THE METHYLENE BLUE BIBLE

5 IN 1

Revolutionary Treatments for Mitochondrial Dysfunction and All Diseases | Unlock the Potential of Methylene Blue for Overall Well-being

Alfred Mallin

© Copyright 2024 - All rights reserved.

The content contained within this book may not be reproduced, duplicated, or transmitted without direct written permission from the author or the publisher.

Under no circumstances will any blame or legal responsibility be held against the publisher, or author, for any damages, reparation, or monetary loss due to the information contained within this book. Either directly or indirectly.

Legal Notice:

This book is copyright protected. This book is only for personal use. You cannot amend, distribute, sell, use, quote, or paraphrase any part, or the content within this book, without the consent of the author or publisher.

Disclaimer Notice:

By reading this document, the reader agrees that under no circumstances is the author responsible for any losses, direct or indirect, which are incurred as a result of the use of the information contained within this document, including, but not limited to, - errors, omissions, or inaccuracies.

The information contained in this book and its contents is not designed to replace or take the place of any form of medical or professional advice; and is not meant to replace the need for independent medical, financial, legal or other professional advice or services, as may be required. The content and information in this book have been provided for educational and entertainment purposes only.

TABLE OF CONTENTS

INTRODUCTION 1

BOOK 1: UNDERSTANDING MITOCHONDRIAL HEALTH 3

Chapter 1: Mitochondrial Health 4
Function and importance 4
Common Dysfunction Causes 5
Cellular Energy Production 6
Role Of Antioxidants 7
Impact Of Aging 8

Chapter 2: Diseases Treated by Mitochondrial Dysfunction 10
Neurodegenerative Diseases 10
Metabolic Disorders 12
Cardiovascular Health 13
Immune System Support 14
Mental Health Conditions 15

BOOK 2: THE SCIENCE BEHIND METHYLENE BLUE 17

Chapter 3: Methylene Blue Overview 18
Historical Use 18
Mechanism of Action 19
Health Benefits 20
Safe Dosages 21
Toxicity Concerns 22

Chapter 4: Revolutionary Treatments Using Methylene Blue 24
Clinical Evidence 24
Dosage Guidelines 25
Combination With Other Treatments 26
Long-Term Use 27
Personalized Treatment Plans 28

BOOK 3: METHYLENE BLUE FOR DISEASE TREATMENT 31

Chapter 5: Diseases Treated by Methylene Blue 32
Neurodegenerative Diseases 32
Metabolic Disorders 33

    Cardiovascular Health 34

    Immune System Support 35

    Mental Health Conditions 36

Chapter 6: Revolutionary Treatment Protocols 38

    Dosage for Various Diseases 38

    Combination Therapies 39

    Treatment Timelines 40

    Case Studies and Patient Stories 41

    Monitoring Health Improvements 43

BOOK 4: PROTOCOLS FOR WELL-BEING 45

Chapter 7: Revolutionary Treatment Protocols 46

    Personalized Treatment Plans 46

    Dosage Guidelines for General Well-Being 48

    Long-Term Methylene Blue Usage 49

    Monitoring Progress and Adjustments 50

    Integrating Methylene Blue with Other Supplements 51

Chapter 8: Integrating Methylene Blue for Well-being 54

    Daily Routines 54

    Nutrition And Supplementation 55

    Preventative Health Strategies 56

    Exercise And Lifestyle Factors 57

    Stress Management 59

BOOK 5: PREVENTATIVE AND LIFESTYLE CARE 61

Chapter 9: Preventative Health Strategies 62

    Importance Of Preventative Care 62

    Building A Healthy Lifestyle Foundation 63

    Routine Health Screenings 65

    Nutritional Strategies for Disease Prevention 66

    Role Of Environmental Factors in Health 67

Chapter 10: Lifestyle for Optimal Mitochondrial Health 69

    Exercise Routines 69

    Reducing Oxidative Stress 70

    Long-Term Care for Aging 71

    Avoiding Toxins and Harmful Habits 72

    Mental And Emotional Wellness 73

Conclusion 75

INTRODUCTION

In recent years, health enthusiasts and medical experts have united in their quest to uncover revolutionary treatments that promise improved health and vitality. *"The Methylene Blue Bible"* stands at the forefront of this exploration, offering a comprehensive guide to one such promising treatment: methylene blue. This book provides an in-depth exploration of its potential, especially in addressing mitochondrial dysfunction—a foe often blamed for a plethora of ailments that plague modern society.

At the heart of cellular energy lies the mitochondria, often referred to as the powerhouses of our cells. These critical organelles are responsible for producing the energy our bodies need to function optimally. However, when they do not perform up to par due to damage or dysfunction, they can be linked to various diseases ranging from neurodegenerative diseases and metabolic disorders to cardiovascular problems and beyond. Hence, understanding and maintaining mitochondrial health becomes paramount for anyone seeking vibrant health.

Methylene blue emerges as an exciting player in this context. Known for its historical use as a dye and medication, it has gained attention within scientific circles for its unique mechanism of action that targets the cellular level. This involves enhancing electron transfer in mitochondria, thereby potentially boosting overall cellular energy production, while offering antioxidative properties that shield cells from oxidative stress—a significant aging factor.

In this book's pages, you will discover how research supports methylene blue's ability to manage and ameliorate symptoms associated with a variety of health conditions. Clinical evidence presented will guide you through dosage considerations, ensuring safe use without toxicity concerns for maximum benefit.

More than just a scientific exposition, *"The Methylene Blue Bible"* brings these findings into practical application across five comprehensive segments: understanding mitochondrial health, diving into the science behind methylene blue, discussing its implication in disease treatment, providing protocols for well-being enhancement, and recommending lifestyle changes for preventative care. Each section is carefully crafted to offer insights that cater to both individuals facing specific health challenges and those with a proactive mindset towards wellness.

Beyond methods and mechanisms lies real stories—case studies and personal journeys that depict methylene blue's transformative effects on lives plagued by conditions like Alzheimer's Disease or Chronic Fatigue Syndrome. These narratives offer readers hope and inspiration by portraying tangible improvements.

Adopting methylene blue as part of one's wellness regimen doesn't operate in isolation; it complements other lifestyle adjustments like nutrition optimization and strategic exercise routines essential for maintaining optimal mitochondrial functionality. Our discussion extends into stress management techniques integral in fostering mental resilience—yet another building block on your path toward holistic health.

"The Methylene Blue Bible" thus serves as an invaluable resource not only for sufferers seeking relief but also for anyone dedicated to understanding their body better—empowering readers with knowledge about cutting-edge therapies that are shaping modern medicine's future landscape.

With every turn of the page comes fresh clarity on how to empower yourself through informed choices concerning treatment options tailored specifically towards achieving optimal health outcomes using methylene blue's extraordinary capabilities.

BOOK 1
UNDERSTANDING MITOCHONDRIAL HEALTH

CHAPTER 1
MITOCHONDRIAL HEALTH

Function and importance

Mitochondria are often referred to as the **powerhouses of the cell**. This is because they produce energy that fuels nearly every cellular process. But there's so much more to learn about them beyond energy production, such as their integral role in maintaining our health.

One of the key functions of mitochondria is regulating cellular metabolism—essentially how cells transform nutrients into usable energy. While we won't dive deep into energy production here, it's important to note that healthy mitochondria ensure effective metabolic processes. This helps maintain a balance between what our cells consume and what they expend.

Mitochondria also controls the life cycle of cells, including their growth and death. This function is critical because it helps our body get rid of old, damaged, or unnecessary cells, making way for fresh and functional ones. Such cellular turnover supports tissue maintenance and overall health.

Beyond their roles within individual cells, mitochondria also assist in communication between cells. They release signals that can influence everything from inflammation responses to cellular repair mechanisms. By facilitating this intercellular communication, mitochondria help maintain harmony within tissues and throughout the immune system.

Another vital aspect of mitochondrial function is calcium storage. Calcium ions serve numerous cellular processes, including muscle contraction and neurotransmitter release, which are essential for brain function and movement coordination. Proper calcium storage by mitochondria ensures these systems have a reliable supply when needed.

In recent years, researchers have also discovered that mitochondria can manage stress responses within the cell. When cells encounter environmental stresses like toxins or high energy demand, mitochondria help to modulate responses and protect cellular structures from damage.

If our mitochondria aren't functioning optimally, it can lead to numerous issues ranging from fatigue to more severe health complications. Researchers study many approaches for supporting mitochondrial health—nutrition being an influential one among them. For clarity on how mitochondrial health impacts general wellness, consider the following simple table highlighting some key mitochondrial functions:

FUNCTION	IMPORTANCE
Energy Metabolism	Fuels cellular activities
Cell Lifecycle Regulation	Assists in cell growth and removal of damaged cells
Intercellular Communication	Influences immune responses and tissue repair
Calcium Storage	Supports muscle contractions and neurotransmission
Stress Management	Helps protect against environmental damage

Understanding these functions helps guide us toward treatments that improve mitochondrial performance for better health outcomes. Remember, embracing a positive relationship with our powerhouse partners enhances not only day-to-day living but also supports us in facing broader health challenges life may throw our way!

Common Dysfunction Causes

As a medical researcher focused on mitochondrial health and alternative treatments, my work often delves into the fundamental causes of mitochondrial dysfunction. The mitochondria, as many of you may know, play a crucial role in cellular health by converting nutrients into usable energy for the cell. When these tiny organelles are disrupted in any way, it can lead to significant health issues. Therefore, understanding the causes of mitochondrial dysfunction is essential.

One major cause of mitochondrial dysfunction is **genetic mutations**. These mutations can occur in either the nuclear DNA or the mitochondrial DNA (mtDNA). Mitochondria have their own DNA, separate from the nuclear DNA found in the cell's nucleus. Mutations in mtDNA can be inherited from one's mother since mitochondria are passed to offspring through the maternal line. These mutations can result in impaired proteins that fail to function correctly in the mitochondria.

Environmental toxins present another source of danger to mitochondrial health. Chemicals such as pesticides, heavy metals like mercury and lead, and pollutants can all damage mitochondria by creating oxidative stress or directly interfering with mitochondrial processes. This disruption often results in a reduced ability to produce energy efficiently, leaving cells struggling to carry out normal functions.

Poor diet is also a notable factor in mitochondrial dysfunction. A diet high in processed foods and low in essential nutrients deprives mitochondria of vital building blocks required for their morning activities. Essential nutrients include vitamins and minerals needed for cofactor functions in enzymatic reactions within the mitochondria.

Furthermore, **metabolic disorders** are linked with mitochondrial issues. Conditions like diabetes can influence how well the mitochondria function. For instance, insulin resistance alters energy production pathways within cells, affecting how glucose is processed and utilized by the mitochondria.

Another point worth mentioning is **stress**—both oxidative stress and physiological stress can be harmful to mitochondria. Oxidative stress results from an imbalance between free radicals and antioxidants in the body, leading to damage at the cellular level. Meanwhile, chronic physiological stress activates pathways that may indirectly damage mitochondrial function over time.

Exposure to certain medications might also lead to mitochondrial damage. Some pharmaceutical drugs interfere with mitochondrial processes either as a side effect or due to unintended interactions with cellular components. Antibiotic use has been documented to harm mitochondria subtly due to similarities between bacterial cells and mitochondria.

Infections also pose risks for mitochondria. Bacterial infections can lead to inflammatory responses that produce reactive oxygen species (ROS), which damage DNA and other cellular structures including those of mitochondria.

By understanding these root causes of mitochondrial dysfunctions, we take steps closer toward identifying effective treatments and preventative measures that maintain optimal cellular activity and support overall well-being for those affected by such conditions.

Cellular Energy Production

To understand energy production, it's essential to look at a process called oxidative phosphorylation. This series of biochemical reactions takes place inside the mitochondria and produces adenosine triphosphate (ATP), the energy currency of our cells. ATP fuels nearly every cell activity, from muscle contraction to neuron signaling.

The process begins with glycolysis, which happens in the cell's cytoplasm, breaking down glucose into pyruvate molecules. These molecules then enter the mitochondria to undergo further transformation through the citric acid cycle, also known as the Krebs cycle.

Within the Krebs cycle, pyruvate is converted into carbon dioxide and high-energy electron carriers like NADH and FADH2. These molecules are fed into the electron transport chain (ETC), a key player in oxidative phosphorylation.

The ETC comprises a series of protein complexes located within the inner mitochondrial membrane. As electrons move through these complexes, protons (hydrogen ions) are pumped across the mitochondrial membrane, creating an electrochemical gradient known as the proton motive force.

This gradient generates potential energy—comparable to water held behind a dam—that is harnessed by ATP synthase, an enzyme that synthesizes ATP from adenosine diphosphate (ADP) and inorganic phosphate. The completion of this cycle results in the production of around 32 molecules of ATP for every glucose molecule processed.

PROCESS	LOCATION	KEY OUTPUTS
Glycolysis	Cytoplasm	Pyruvate + small amounts of ATP
Krebs Cycle	Mitochondrial matrix	CO2 + NADH + FADH2
Electron Transport Chain	Inner mitochondrial membrane	Large amounts of ATP

It's important to note that this complex yet efficient system is susceptible to various challenges. Factors such as genetic mutations, environmental toxins, and lifestyle choices can disrupt mitochondrial function. When any part of this process falters, it can lead to reduced ATP production and contribute to mitochondrial dysfunction—a condition implicated in numerous diseases ranging from metabolic disorders to neurodegenerative diseases.

In my exploration of alternative treatments, I've delved into various compounds believed to support mitochondrial health and enhance energy production. Among these substances is methylene blue, which has shown promise in preliminary studies for its potential role in facilitating electron transport within mitochondria. Methylene blue may help bypass damaged complexes in the ETC, ensuring continued ATP production even when some parts suffer impairment.

While more research is needed to fully understand its mechanisms and efficacy thoroughly, investigating treatments like methylene blue offers hope for addressing mitochondrial dysfunction at its root—at the vital level of energy production within our cells. This ongoing research endeavors not only aspire to enhance longevity but also improve quality of life by supporting one's cellular machinery.

Role Of Antioxidants

Mitochondria are vulnerable to damage from free radicals, which are unstable molecules that can harm cellular components. Antioxidants protects mitochondria from oxidative stress, thereby preserving their function and enhancing overall cellular health.

One of the primary roles of antioxidants is to neutralize free radicals. These free radicals are by-products of normal biochemical processes in the body, including those that occur during energy production within the mitochondria. Left unchecked, these rogue molecules can lead to a state known as oxidative stress, which damages cellular structures, including DNA, proteins, and lipids. This damage can result in mitochondrial dysfunction, contributing to various diseases.

Vitamin E and vitamin C are key antioxidant vitamins that help combat oxidative stress. Vitamin E is a fat-soluble vitamin, meaning it plays a protective role within the lipid-rich environments of cell membranes. By scavenging free radicals, vitamin E helps prevent lipid peroxidation—a process where free radicals steal electrons from the lipids in cell membranes, leading to cell damage. Meanwhile, vitamin C is a water-soluble antioxidant that works primarily in the aqueous compartments of cells and tissues. It regenerates vitamin E and can directly neutralize different types of free radicals.

In addition to these vitamins, there are several other potent antioxidants such as glutathione and coenzyme Q10 (CoQ10). Glutathione is often referred to as the "master antioxidant" due to its presence in high concentrations within cells and its role in recycling other antioxidants back to their active forms. It's vital for detoxification processes as well as maintaining immune function. Similarly, CoQ10 is naturally produced by the body and concentrated in the mitochondria. It's essential for energy production and also serves an important antioxidant role by protecting mitochondrial membranes from oxidative damage.

There is evidence suggesting that antioxidant supplementation may improve mitochondrial function. For instance, CoQ10 supplements have been shown to enhance energy production and reduce fatigue in people with mitochondrial disorders. Moreover, certain polyphenols like resveratrol found in grapes have been noted for their potential benefits on mitochondrial health through their antioxidant properties.

It's essential to address that while antioxidants have significant protective benefits for mitochondria, balance is key; excessive consumption or inappropriate supplementation can sometimes be counterproductive or even harmful. Thus, it is ideal to obtain antioxidants through a balanced diet rich in fruits, vegetables, nuts, and seeds rather than relying solely on supplements.

Incorporating these nutrients into our diet provides a natural synergy of compounds that work together to enhance antioxidant capacity more effectively than isolated nutrients might achieve alone.

ANTIOXIDANT	SOURCES	BENEFITS
Vitamin E	Nuts (almonds), seeds (sunflower)	Protects cell membranes

Vitamin C	Citrus fruits (oranges), berries	Neutralizes free radicals
Glutathione	Garlic, onions	Detoxification and immune system support
CoQ10	Nuts (almonds), seeds (sunflower)	Energy production and mitochondrial protection
Resveratrol	Grapes, red wine	Potential mitochondrial health benefits

While research continues to uncover more about these powerful agents' intricacies and their interactions with cellular processes, it's clear that they offer promising avenues for defending our cells against oxidative damage while supporting overall vitality.

Impact Of Aging

It's undeniable that as we age, our cells gradually lose their youthful vigor, and much of this decline is intricately linked to mitochondrial function. You see, our mitochondria are responsible for producing the energy necessary for nearly every cellular process. With age, however, their efficiency tends to wane.

The process of aging impacts mitochondria in several significant ways. One major factor is the accumulation of mutations in mitochondrial DNA (mtDNA). Unlike nuclear DNA, mtDNA does not enjoy the same robust repair mechanisms, resulting in these mutations accruing over time. These genetic alterations can impair mitochondrial function, hindering energy production and contributing to the overall decline in cellular function that we observe as aging progresses.

Another consequence of aging on mitochondrial health is a reduction in mitochondrial biogenesis—the process by which new mitochondria are produced. This decline means that older cells may operate with fewer functional mitochondria, thus exacerbating energy deficits and potentially leading to a variety of age-related ailments.

Aging also influences the dynamic processes of fusion and fission within mitochondria. These processes are crucial as they allow mitochondria to maintain their functionality by adapting to cellular requirements and stressors. With age-related stressors increasing, the balance between these two processes can be disrupted, reducing mitochondrial quality control and their ability to effectively respond to metabolic demands.

Oxidative stress becomes more pronounced with age as well. While mitochondria are a primary source of reactive oxygen species (ROS), they are also targets for oxidative damage. As we age, excess ROS levels can overwhelm antioxidant defenses, leading to damage not only within mitochondria but also throughout various cellular structures—further accelerating the decline in cellular integrity.

Let's take a look at how these changes manifest in more tangible terms through some studies conducted over the years:

PHENOMENON	IMPACT ON MITOCHONDRIAL HEALTH
mtDNA Mutation Accumulation	Energy production declines due to impaired genes
Decreased Mitochondrial Biogenesis	Reduced cellular energy availability
Imbalance in Fusion/Fission	Compromised ability to manage metabolic demands
Increased Oxidative Stress	Accelerated damage affecting cell functions

What does all this mean for us as individuals seeking healthier aging? It underscores the importance of targeting mitochondria if we aim for enhanced longevity. A promising area I've been exploring involves interventions such as dietary regulations—caloric restriction in particular shows promise by potentially boosting mitochondrial efficiency and reducing oxidative stress.

Moreover, particular supplements have shown potential benefits for aging mitochondria. Coenzyme Q10, often discussed in scientific circles due its essential role in electron transport chain function, is one supplement that might help counteract some deficiencies associated with aging. Additionally, agents like Methylene Blue have been researched for their potential small-scale effects on electron flow in mitochondria. Understanding how aging influences our mitochondria opens pathways to groundbreaking treatments that could revolutionize how we perceive healthspan and lifespan.

CHAPTER 2
DISEASES TREATED BY MITOCHONDRIAL DYSFUNCTION

Neurodegenerative Diseases

While the role of mitochondria has been discussed, let's focus on its implications in neurological health, specifically concerning diseases like Alzheimer's, Parkinson's, and Huntington's disease. Neurodegenerative diseases are conditions that result in the progressive degeneration or death of nerve cells, causing problems with movement (ataxias) or mental functioning (dementias).

Current research is increasingly pointing towards mitochondrial dysfunction as a key factor in the development and progression of these diseases. The mitochondria are responsible for producing energy in our cells through a process called oxidative phosphorylation. When this function is compromised, it can lead to cell damage and death.

Alzheimer's Disease

Alzheimer's disease is the most common neurodegenerative disorder, characterized by memory loss and cognitive decline. Research has shown a significant link between impaired mitochondrial function and Alzheimer's. In this context, I'm particularly interested in how supporting mitochondrial health might slow down or prevent the onset of such symptoms. The accumulation of defective mitochondria leads to increased oxidative stress—a harmful process that further damages cells. This oxidative stress is believed to play a critical role in Alzheimer's pathology.

By targeting mitochondrial dysfunction, we aim to enhance healthy aging processes and improve energy metabolism within brain cells. This approach holds promise not only for slowing disease progression but also for potentially reversing some degree of neuronal damage.

Parkinson's Disease

Parkinson's disease primarily affects movement, often starting with tremors that eventually lead to rigidity and bradykinesia—or slowness of movement. In Parkinson's patients, studies indicate a relapse into energy failure due to impaired mitochondrial complex I activity within the cells that produce dopamine—a neurotransmitter crucial for coordinating movement.

The inability to maintain proper function results in neuronal loss predominantly in the substantia nigra region of the brain. By focusing on improving mitochondrial efficiency, we can enhance dopaminergic neuron survival rates and thus alleviate some motor symptoms associated with Parkinson's disease.

Huntington's Disease

Huntington's disease presents another case where mitochondrial dysfunction plays a critical role—it causes uncontrolled movements and emotional disturbances brought about by genetic mutations leading to neurotoxicity. These mutations disrupt normal cellular functions including mitochondrial respiration and energy production.

Mitochondrial support therapies aim at enhancing cell resilience by counteracting these detrimental effects—improving both cognitive abilities and quality of life for individuals affected by Huntington's disease.

Therapies Targeting Mitochondrial Dysfunction

Several therapeutic strategies have emerged aimed at protecting neurons from degeneration through optimal mitochondrial function:

1. **Antioxidant supplementation:** Antioxidants help reduce oxidative stress levels within neurons.
2. **Mitochondrial biogenesis activators:** Compounds like resveratrol promote the creation of new mitochondria.
3. **Targeted drug therapy:** Drugs such as Methylene Blue have shown promise due to their ability to enhance cellular respiration directly at mitochondria sites.

Within emerging treatments rooted in addressing mitochondrial dysfunction, two significant modalities stand out:

1. **Nutritional Approaches:** A diet rich in antioxidants and supportive nutrients can be integral in bolstering mitochondrial function. Nutrients such as Coenzyme Q10 and Omega-3 fatty acids have been shown to support cellular energy production. Further, diet adjustments focusing on caloric restriction or ketosis may promote mitochondrial efficiency, offering new avenues for intervention.
2. **Lifestyle Modifications:** Regular physical exercise is known to stimulate mitochondrial biogenesis, improving overall mitochondrial function. By encouraging neuronal health and plasticity, exercise could serve as a foundational element of preventative strategies against neurodegenerative diseases.

In my work, I've examined various interventions like these not only for their standalone benefits but also their synergistic effects when combined with pharmacological treatments. This integrated approach paves the way for comprehensive therapies that target not just the symptoms but underlying mitochondrial dysfunction in neurodegenerative diseases.

INTERVENTION TYPE	POTENTIAL BENEFIT
Antioxidant supplementation	Reduces oxidative stress within neurons
Mitochondrial biogenesis activators	Promotes creation of new mitochondria

Targeted drug therapy	Enhances cellular respiration at mitochondria
Nutritional approaches	Supports cellular energy production
Lifestyle modifications	Stimulates mitochondrial function

Metabolic Disorders

Mitochondrial dysfunction often leads to insufficient ATP production, the energy currency essential for numerous biochemical reactions. This inadequacy can drive or exacerbate metabolic disorders such as diabetes, obesity, and inherited syndromes like Leigh syndrome or MELAS syndrome (Mitochondrial Encephalopathy, Lactic Acidosis, and Stroke-like episodes). In diabetes, for instance, impaired mitochondrial function can alter insulin sensitivity and glucose metabolism. Similarly, mitochondrial abnormalities in obesity may impede effective lipid metabolism, leading to excessive fat accumulation.

Another noteworthy aspect is how mitochondrial dysfunction contributes to lipotoxicity — a condition where excess fatty acids and their metabolites initiate harmful effects on organs not primarily involved in fat storage. This phenomenon is closely observed in conditions like non-alcoholic fatty liver disease (NAFLD), where an overload of fat in liver cells triggers inflammation and insulin resistance.

From personal research and clinical observation, it's clear that addressing mitochondrial health could significantly impact these conditions. By improving mitochondrial function through lifestyle interventions or therapeutic agents like Coenzyme Q10 or Methylene Blue—a topic deeply explored within this book—we can enhance energy efficiency and manage symptoms better.

The efficacy of Methylene Blue specifically lies in its ability to act as an electron donor during impaired cellular respiration, theoretically bypassing damaged complexes in the electron transport chain. This capacity makes it a promising candidate for improving outcomes in patients with mitochondrial-linked metabolic disorders.

METABOLIC DISORDER	MITOCHONDRIAL ROLE	POTENTIAL THERAPEUTIC APPROACHES
Diabetes	Impaired glucose/insulin regulation	Improved diet/exercise, Metformin, Coenzyme Q10
Obesity	Lipid oxidation inefficiency	Weight management programs, lifestyle interventions
Non-Alcoholic Fatty Liver Disease	Lipotoxicity and oxidative stress	Dietary changes, pharmaceutical interventions (e.g., antioxidants)
Leigh Syndrome	Energy production deficits	Supportive therapies (nutritional supplementation)
MELAS Syndrome	Faulty electron transport	Vitamins/co-factors (e.g., L-carnitine), Methylene Blue

In understanding these associations and potential treatment strategies better, we open doors for more personalized interventions that account for individual variations in mitochondrial function. This approach signals a paradigm shift—focusing not just on symptom management but also addressing root causes at the cellular level.

As research continues to shed light on the intricate connections between mitochondria and metabolic disorders, it becomes increasingly feasible to develop targeted therapies that alleviate symptoms and improve quality of life for those affected by these challenging conditions.

Cardiovascular Health

Cardiovascular diseases remain a leading cause of death globally. They include conditions such as coronary artery disease, heart failure, and hypertension. Mitochondria, being the powerhouse of our cells, have long been considered key players in maintaining heart health. When they don't function correctly, it can lead to various cardiovascular issues.

It's essential to grasp how mitochondria are implicated in these diseases. In healthy hearts, mitochondria produce vast amounts of energy necessary for the continuous pumping of blood. This energy production involves the process we know as oxidative phosphorylation. However, when this process is disrupted—due to genetic mutations, aging, or lifestyle factors—the efficiency of mitochondrial energy production decreases.

One major consequence of poor mitochondrial function is the imbalance between energy supply and demand in heart cells. When energy demands exceed what these faulty mitochondria can supply, it leads to ischemic conditions. Ischemia refers to insufficient blood supply to tissues, causing oxygen deprivation. In the heart, this is one pathway toward conditions like angina or even myocardial infarction (heart attack).

Mitochondrial dysfunction is also linked to oxidative stress—a situation where excess free radicals are not adequately neutralized by antioxidants. Free radicals are molecules that can damage cellular components, including lipids, proteins, and DNA within our cells. This situation is particularly harmful for heart cells because they require immense amounts of energy and are highly susceptible to oxidative damage.

Furthermore, studies indicate that dysfunctional mitochondria release signals that can trigger apoptosis (programmed cell death). Apoptosis in cardiac cells can weaken heart tissue over time and contribute significantly to heart failure.

Exploring treatment possibilities takes us to promising alternatives like methylene blue—a compound that exhibits potential benefits in addressing mitochondrial dysfunctions due to its unique properties enhancing mitochondrial respiration.

CONDITION	PROPER MITOCHONDRIAL FUNCTION	IMPAIRED MITOCHONDRIAL FUNCTION
Energy Supply	Adequate ATP production ensures optimal heart ability	Reduced ATP leads to insufficient heart exertion
Oxidative Stress	Balanced ROS formation; efficient antioxidant defenses	Excessive ROS; insufficient antioxidant protection
Cellular Health	Designed apoptosis occurs naturally and healthily	Increased apoptosis damages tissue integrity

Such a table paints a clear picture: proper mitochondrial function is vital for sustaining cardiovascular health. Emerging therapies targeting mitochondrial dysfunction offer hope for novel treatments aimed at strengthening cardiovascular function naturally or via medications like methylene blue. Our understanding continues to grow with every study published.

Immune System Support

The immune system is our body's defense mechanism against infections and diseases. It relies on energy to attack and neutralize harmful invaders like bacteria and viruses. This is where mitochondria play a starring role. They provide the energy needed for immune cells to perform their tasks efficiently. When mitochondrial function is impaired, it's akin to trying to protect a fortress with a weakened army—our defenses become less effective.

Mitochondrial dysfunction can lead to an impaired immune response in several ways. It can cause reduced production of ATP (the primary energy currency of the cell), leading to fatigued immune cells that aren't up to the task of warding off infections. Furthermore, malfunctioning mitochondria may inadvertently produce excessive reactive oxygen species (ROS), which can damage cells, including those that make up our immune system.

KEY COMPONENT	ROLE IN IMMUNE SYSTEM	MITOCHONDRIAL IMPACT
ATP Production	Powers immune cell functions	Reduced production hampers cell activity
Reactive Oxygen Species (ROS)	Signals for launching defense mechanisms	Excessive ROS causes cell damage and weakens immunity

One area where this connection becomes apparent is in chronic fatigue syndrome (CFS), which has garnered attention partly due to its mysterious origins and debilitating symptoms. Many researchers, including myself, believe that mitochondrial dysfunction plays a role in CFS by compromising immune function. Individuals with CFS often have low ATP levels and oxidative stress markers, aligning with our understanding of mitochondrial impairment's role.

The exciting development here is that supporting mitochondrial function could boost immune health and even assist in treating diseases linked with mitochondrial dysfunction. One tool that has emerged as particularly promising is methylene blue. It acts as an electron cycler within mitochondria, improving their efficiency and potentially restoring energy balance in the body.

In our discussions on revolutionary treatments for mitochondrial dysfunction, methylene blue stands out not only for its ability to enhance cellular energy but also for its potential in supporting immune system resilience. Although more research is needed to fully harness its capabilities across various diseases, early evidence suggests it's a simple yet powerful molecule deserving attention.

From my experience and ongoing studies, taking steps toward optimizing mitochondrial health can lead to significant benefits across the board—including better immune function. Lifestyle factors such as a balanced diet rich in antioxidants, regular physical activity (tailored to individual capacity), and managing stress levels all support healthy mitochondria.

Incorporating nutritional supplements shown to benefit mitochondrial activity could also play a role here. Coenzyme Q10 and B vitamins are examples supported by research in enhancing cellular energetics and reducing oxidative damage—which together strengthen both mitochondria and immunity.

The intersection between mitochondrial health and immunity opens intriguing avenues not just for treatment but proactive wellness strategies too. Whether tackling a specific condition or preserving long-term health, this holistic view reminds us how interconnected systems work best when fundamental processes like energy production are optimized.

Mental Health Conditions

In recent years, there's been growing evidence that mitochondrial dysfunction is linked to several mental health disorders. The connection is fascinating yet complex, like piecing together a puzzle where each discovery brings us closer to seeing the bigger picture of mental wellness.

Let's start with depression, one of the most common mental health disorders worldwide. Research suggests that when mitochondria are not functioning optimally, it may lead to the brain not getting enough energy. This energy deficiency can then contribute to symptoms of depression. Imagine your brain feeling tired and sluggish because every cell is running on low battery power. Without enough energy, it's hard for the brain to regulate mood and respond effectively to stress.

Interestingly, studies have shown that traditional antidepressants might influence mitochondrial function. Some researchers are even exploring treatments specifically targeting mitochondria to alleviate depression symptoms more effectively. It's an exciting frontier that could provide new hope for those who haven't found relief through conventional medications.

Schizophrenia is another condition where mitochondrial dysfunction plays a critical role. The exact causes of schizophrenia are still not completely understood, but it appears that impaired mitochondrial function may contribute to the development of this disorder. Mitochondria are crucial for neuron survival and synaptic plasticity—the brain's ability to adapt and reorganize itself—which are often disrupted in schizophrenia.

Bipolar disorder also seems to be closely linked with mitochondrial issues. In bipolar disorder, mood swings range from manic highs to depressive lows, and these shifts might be related to how well mitochondria can respond to cellular stress throughout different phases of this cycle. Researchers have found that individuals with bipolar disorder often show alterations in genes related to mitochondrial function, suggesting a strong link between the two.

Anxiety disorders represent yet another area where mitochondrial dysfunction seems influential. Anxiety can be incredibly draining on both mind and body, leaving one feeling perpetually on edge or tense without clear reason. This chronic stress state demands a lot from our mitochondria since they need to keep generating ample energy for prolonged periods under duress—a task they might struggle with if already compromised.

Emerging research indicates that improving mitochondrial efficiency could potentially ease anxiety symptoms by reducing cellular stress levels overall. Therapeutic strategies aimed at enhancing mitochondrial health are being considered alternatives or adjuncts alongside more established anxiety interventions like therapy or medication.

MENTAL HEALTH CONDITION	ROLE OF MITOCHONDRIAL DYSFUNCTION

Depression	Energy deficiency affecting mood regulation
Schizophrenia	Impaired neuron viability and synaptic plasticity
Bipolar Disorder	Alterations in stress response mechanisms during mood shifts
Anxiety Disorders	Insufficient energy production leading exacerbated stress response

While more research is needed before we fully understand all these interactions and how best they can be harnessed therapeutically, one thing remains clear—our mitochondria play an essential role when it comes to maintaining mental health resilience over time.

The knowledge we've gathered so far signifies promising advancements looming horizon beyond traditional treatment paradigms alone: namely ones focusing upon strengthening fundamental cellular bioenergetics underpinning psychiatric wellness thereby augmenting broader physical resilience simultaneously—a truly integrated holistic approach beneficial across board!

BOOK 2
THE SCIENCE BEHIND METHYLENE BLUE

CHAPTER 3
METHYLENE BLUE OVERVIEW

Historical Use

Methylene blue is a compound that might sound unusual at first, but it's been around for quite a long time, and its story is truly fascinating. As someone who is deeply interested in mitochondrial health and alternative treatments, I find the history of methylene blue to be both intriguing and enlightening. Methylene blue was first synthesized in 1876 by Heinrich Caro, a German chemist. Originally, it was developed as a dye for textiles due to its vibrant blue color. However, it wasn't long before its potential medicinal properties were discovered, opening new avenues for its use.

Historically, one of the earliest medical applications of methylene blue dates back to the late 19th century. It was used as a treatment for malaria, a severe disease caused by parasites transmitted through mosquito bites. Researchers found that methylene blue could effectively target the malaria parasite within red blood cells. While other more effective antimalarial drugs were developed later on, methylene blue paved the way for understanding how synthetic chemicals could intervene in parasitic diseases.

The early 20th century saw methylene blue being used as a diagnostic aid and treatment in other areas of medicine too. Its ability to stain tissues made it valuable in identifying certain medical conditions. For instance, surgeons utilized it during surgical procedures to better visualize specific areas of tissue. Moreover, it was employed in tests to diagnose urinary tract infections because when consumed orally, methylene blue would color the urine if it encountered an alkaline substance.

Interestingly enough, methylene blue played a part in psychiatry as well. Around the 1890s, some psychiatrists explored its effects on mental health conditions like schizophrenia and bipolar disorder. While our understanding and treatment approaches have advanced significantly since then, these early attempts highlighted methylene blue's potential impact on brain chemistry.

The varying uses of methylene blue can be seen as stepping stones that have broadened its application scope over time. In recent decades, interest in this compound has been renewed thanks to emerging research indicating its potential benefits for mitochondrial function. This avenue of study holds promise because mitochondria are vital components within our cells responsible for producing energy.

In this overview of historical uses of methylene blue, one thing becomes clear: each step in its journey has contributed insights into how substances could interact with biological systems to yield therapeutic outcomes. Whether aiding diagnosis or offering treatment pathways during times when modern medicine had yet to unfold its myriad options—we owe much credit to pioneers who ventured into uncharted territories using this remarkable substance.

To encapsulate the evolution from textile dye invention through multifaceted roles across different medical fields, methylene blue's story underscores how innovations can sometimes arise from unexpected origins—an intriguing thought that leaves me pondering what other hidden gems might lie in waiting amidst today's research landscapes!

TIMELINE	USE	DESCRIPTION
1876	Textile Dye	First synthesized for dyeing fabrics thanks to its brilliant hue
Late 1800s	Malaria Treatment	Early antimalarial drug targeting parasites inside red blood cells
	Psychiatry	Experimented with effects on mental health disorders (schizophrenia/bipolar)
Early 1900s	Diagnostic Aid/Urinary Tract Infection Tests	Utilized due to staining properties; confirmed infections via colored urine changes

This table reflects not only chronological developments but also highlights versatility inherent within seemingly simple compounds like methylene blue—a lesson ever relevant while exploring potentials nestled within scientific endeavors!

Mechanism of Action

Methylene Blue is a synthetic compound that has been in use for over a century. Initially synthesized as a dye, MB has transitioned into the medical realm due to its unique properties. At its core, MB acts as an electron cycler. This means it can accept and donate electrons, crucial players in the cellular energy game.

To understand Methylene Blue's mechanism of action, let's take a step back and look at cellular respiration. Imagine your cells as factories. The mitochondria are like power plants in these factories, producing the energy currency, ATP (adenosine triphosphate), which powers various cellular processes. Within these mitochondria, there's a biochemical process known as the electron transport chain (ETC), which plays a fundamental role in energy production.

When the electron transport chain faces disruptions—due to factors like oxidative stress or dysfunctional components—energy production can slow down or even halt. MB can step in to facilitate this process. By shuttling electrons through its structure, MB helps bypass blockages within the ETC. This means it can essentially "*unclog*" and aid in the smooth flow of electrons, ensuring continued ATP production even under stress.

Another aspect of MB's action is its antioxidant capability. Amid oxidative stress—where harmful free radicals threaten cell components—MB acts like a buffer. It neutralizes these free radicals before they can wreak havoc on cellular structures. In doing so, it preserves mitochondrial function and integrity.

It's also worth noting how Methylene Blue interacts with nitric oxide (NO). While NO is vital for cellular functions like maintaining vascular health, excessive amounts can impair mitochondrial function. Methylene Blue can bind to NO, inhibiting its overproduction. This regulation helps maintain normal cellular operations without tipping into harmful territory.

ELECTRON TRANSPORT CHAIN	OXIDATIVE STRESS	NITRIC OXIDE INTERACTIONS
Accepts/donates electrons to bypass blockages	Neutralizes free radicals to protect cells	Binds to excess NO to prevent mitochondrial inhibition
Supports consistent ATP production	Acts as an antioxidizing agent	Stabilizes NO levels for balanced function

Methylene Blue's capabilities extend beyond these points; however, these functions highlight why it's considered in studies involving brain health and other areas impacted by mitochondrial dysfunction. Its role as an electron donor/acceptor provides critical support during energy production challenges within our cells' powerhouses—the mitochondria.

Health Benefits

Methylene Blue is not just a dye used in laboratories; it's a compound with promising health benefits that could be instrumental in revolutionizing treatments for mitochondrial dysfunction.

Every cell in our body contains mitochondria, churning away like tiny engines converting nutrients into energy. When these engines malfunction, it's not difficult to imagine the cascade of issues that can arise. This is where Methylene Blue steps in—a molecule that has shown potential as a therapeutic agent by improving mitochondrial function.

Here's what the research tells us so far:

1. **Energy Boost and Mental Clarity:** Methylene Blue has been shown to act as an electron cycler. Essentially, it helps shuttle electrons back and forth within the mitochondria, aiding in energy production. You might think of it like an extra hand on a conveyor belt, ensuring things move smoothly and efficiently. This increased efficiency can translate into enhanced cognitive function and mental clarity. Imagine switching from a dial-up connection to high-speed Internet—everything just works better.

2. **Neuroprotection:** One of the most exciting areas of research involves Methylene Blue's neuroprotective properties. Studies have demonstrated that it can protect neurons from damage caused by oxidative stress—a major contributor to neurodegenerative diseases like Alzheimer's and Parkinson's. By reducing oxidative stress, Methylene Blue helps maintain healthier brain cells, which supports better memory retention and cognitive function.

3. **Anti-inflammatory Effects:** Chronic inflammation is at the heart of many modern ailments, from arthritis to heart disease. Research indicates that Methylene Blue has anti-inflammatory properties, which could help reduce inflammation throughout the body. Not only does

this alleviate pain and discomfort associated with inflammation, but it also tackles one of its root causes, potentially slowing disease progression.

4. **Antimicrobial Properties:** Methylene Blue doesn't just target human cells; it's also effective against harmful bacteria and parasites without wreaking havoc on beneficial microbes within our systems. In fact, it has been used historically as a treatment for malaria due to its ability to interfere with parasitic cell division.

To visualize its potential impact on mitochondrial function—notably energy production—I've included a simple table showcasing how Methylene Blue compares to other common interventions:

INTERVENTION	MECHANISM	EFFECT ON ENERGY PRODUCTION
Methylene Blue	Electron cycling	High efficiency improvement
CoQ10 Supplement	Electron chain support	Moderate support
Vitamin B Complex	Co-factor supplementation	Supportive but less direct

It's clear from this comparison why there's so much excitement about this compound. While further studies are necessary to fully understand the breadth of its benefits—and indeed best practices for its use—it feels reassuringly like we are just scratching the surface of what may become a groundbreaking component in treating countless diseases rooted in cellular energy dysfunction.

Safe Dosages

It's important to know that methylene blue has been used in medicine for various purposes, often at different dosages depending on the application. For instance, it's been employed as an antidote for certain types of poisoning and as a diagnostic dye with varying amounts necessary for each specific use.

You might be wondering, *what exactly constitutes a safe dosage of Methylene Blue for human use?* When considering methylene blue for supporting mitochondrial health and other potential benefits, dosages can vary. The key here is moderation and personalization based on individual needs and circumstances. In many cases, low doses have been suggested for supportive health purposes. From my experience as a medical researcher focused on mitochondrial health, I've found that individuals often experiment within a broadly accepted range to find what works best for them.

Generally, doses ranging from 0.5 mg/kg to about 4 mg/kg body weight are considered low and potentially beneficial for various applications. These amounts are typically well-tolerated by most people. Here's a simple example: if you weigh 70 kg (about 154 pounds), this means your intake might start as low as 35 mg per day when aiming for lower dosages and could be adjusted upwards gradually as you monitor your response.

Here's a basic table format that illustrates possible dosing based on body weight:

BODY WEIGHT (KG)	LOW DOSE RANGE (MG/DAY)
50	25 - 200
60	30 - 240
70	35 - 280
80	40 - 320
90	45 - 360

Remember, these figures are just guidelines and should be adjusted according to individual tolerance and therapeutic goals. It's also essential to take methylene blue under the guidance of a healthcare professional familiar with its use. Monitoring response is another critical aspect of safe dosing. I always suggest that newcomers start at the lower end of the spectrum to observe how their body reacts before considering any increase in dosage. This approach helps mitigate any potential side effects or unwanted reactions.

Moreover, consistency in dosage timing can improve how well methylene blue works for you. Some people find it beneficial to split their dosage across meals to enhance absorption and maintain stable levels throughout the day. Others may prefer taking it all at once if they find it more convenient or effective based on personal experience.

In some cases, people may cycle their usage of methylene blue — perhaps using it for several weeks followed by a short break — though research on the effectiveness of such an approach is still emerging. While methylene blue has shown promise as an agent supporting mitochondrial health and beyond, correct dosing tailored to your unique needs makes all the difference in leveraging its benefits safely and effectively. If you're considering incorporating methylene blue into your wellness routine, do so thoughtfully and always consult with healthcare providers experienced in this area.

Toxicity Concerns

Like any compound we think about using for health benefits, we also need to understand its potential risks—especially toxicity concerns. Methylene blue has been used in various forms for over a hundred years now. Originally emerging from the textile industry as a dye, it found its way into medicine during the late 19th century. But with its increasing use, questions about its safety started to arise. Despite its promising benefits, methylene blue is subject to scrutiny when it comes to safety profiles—and rightfully so.

Toxicity refers to the harmful effects that may arise from exposure to certain substances like chemicals or medications. In the case of methylene blue, while generally considered safe within prescribed limits, certain factors could lead one to experience adverse effects if not properly managed.

One primary concern with methylene blue is that it can cause hemolytic anemia in individuals who suffer from specific enzyme deficiencies, such as glucose-6-phosphate dehydrogenase (G6PD) deficiency. Without adequate levels of this enzyme, red blood cells become vulnerable when exposed to oxidative stressors like methylene blue. This leads to the premature breakdown of these cells—an occurrence known as hemolysis. For people with G6PD deficiency, special caution needs to be taken regarding methylene blue usage.

Symptoms of such an adverse reaction may include paleness or jaundice (yellowing of the skin), dark urine, and fatigue—all signs that should prompt you to stop usage immediately and seek medical advice.

There are also concerns regarding potential interactions with other medications that affect serotonin levels in the brain—a condition known as serotonin syndrome. When taken alongside medications that increase serotonin activity (such as certain antidepressants), methylene blue may cause excessive accumulation of serotonin in the brain leading to symptoms like confusion, hyperactivity, rapid heart rate, blood pressure changes, or even life-threatening reactions if not addressed promptly.

Moreover, high doses are known to result in bluish discoloration of bodily fluids—like urine or saliva—a harmless yet somewhat startling effect that takes place during treatment with high concentrations.

POTENTIAL TOXICITY CONCERNS	SYMPTOMS/EFFECTS	PRECAUTIONARY MEASURES
Hemolytic anemia (in G6PD deficiency)	Fatigue, jaundice, dark urine	Avoid usage if diagnosed with G6PD deficiency
Serotonin Syndrome	Confusion, altered mental status	Monitor medication interactions (especially antidepressants)
High dose discoloration	Bluish urine/saliva	Understand it's benign; happens on higher doses

But fear not—the good news is that when administered appropriately within recommended dosages by a healthcare professional aware of your individual medical history and concurrent medication intake—methylene blue remains a valuable addition in therapeutic strategies. Despite these challenges linked with toxicity concerns under certain conditions or misuse scenarios—the value brought forth by methylene blue evidently outweighs potential setbacks when handled responsibly.

CHAPTER 4
REVOLUTIONARY TREATMENTS USING METHYLENE BLUE

Clinical Evidence

Methylene blue has long been known for its role as a dye, but its medical uses are becoming incredibly interesting. Over the years, scientists have explored how it can improve mitochondrial function, which is crucial because our mitochondria are like tiny powerhouses within our cells. They produce energy that keeps us alive and well.

Recent studies have shifted attention toward methylene blue's therapeutic potential. For instance, it's being explored extensively for neurodegenerative diseases like Alzheimer's and Parkinson's. Clinical trials suggest that methylene blue may help slow cognitive decline in Alzheimer's patients by improving brain cell function and energy production.

Another exciting area where methylene blue is making waves is in the treatment of mood disorders such as depression and anxiety. Some smaller trials indicate that it may enhance mood by increasing brain energy metabolism. Although larger-scale studies are necessary to fully understand these effects, early results encourage optimism.

Cancer treatment is another field where researchers are investigating the benefits of methylene blue. Some preclinical studies highlight its ability to disrupt cancer cell growth while sparing healthy cells by targeting dysfunctional oxidative processes within malignant cells. This targeted action suggests a promising adjunctive role in oncology.

I want to highlight an interesting study published in recent years. It reported improvements in patients suffering from photophobia — sensitivity to light — using low doses of methylene blue. It appears that this compound can stabilize visual processing pathways, providing relief to those afflicted by this challenging symptom.

One area worth mentioning is its impact on skin health. Methylene blue shows great promise in dermatology by promoting skin repair and reducing scars due to its ability to modulate cellular stress responses effectively.

CONDITION	POTENTIAL BENEFITS	CURRENT STAGE OF RESEARCH
Alzheimer's & Parkinson's	Slows cognitive decline	Ongoing clinical trials
Depression & Anxiety	Enhances mood	Early-stage trials
Cancer	Targets cancer cell growth	Preclinical studies
Photophobia	Reduces light sensitivity	Case reports
Skin Health	Promotes repair, reduces scars	Experimental studies

While all these findings sound promising, it's crucial for anyone interested in this compound's therapeutic potential to stay tuned for further research results and regulatory approvals. The journey from clinical research to everyday clinical practice can be lengthy but worthwhile if successful.

Dosage Guidelines

Methylene blue (MB) has emerged as an innovative therapeutic agent that can support individuals with various health issues, particularly those related to mitochondrial dysfunction. Accurate dosage is crucial to ensure safety and effectiveness. Methylene blue operates on a cellular level, enhancing the efficiency of energy production in our cells. Keeping the dosage right is important because it's a powerful compound. Too little may yield no effect, while too much could lead to unwanted side effects like dizziness or nausea. Typically, dosages can vary based on factors such as age, weight, and specific health conditions. For general guidance:

1. **Low Dose:** 0.5 mg/kg per day – This is generally considered safe for most individuals looking to support cellular metabolism.
2. **Moderate Dose:** 1-2 mg/kg per day – This range might be used by individuals experiencing more significant mitochondrial distress or neurological symptoms.
3. **High Dose:** Above 2 mg/kg per day – Generally reserved for specific cases under professional supervision, especially in research settings.

WEIGHT (KG)	LOW DOSE (MG)	MODERATE DOSE (MG)	HIGH DOSE (MG)
50	25	50-100	100+
60	30	60-120	120+
70	35	70-140	140+
80	40	80-160	160+

This chart provides a quick overview based on different body weights. Adjusting doses for individual circumstances is important.

Guidelines for Optimal Use

1. **Starting Low and Slow:** Begin with the lowest effective dose and gradually adjust upwards if necessary. This approach minimizes the risk of side effects.
2. **Listening to Your Body:** Pay attention to how you feel once you start using methylene blue. If you notice any discomfort or unusual symptoms, consult a healthcare provider promptly.
3. **Timing of Doses:** Consistency is key—take your doses at the same time each day for the best results.
4. **Monitoring Progress:** Some folks might opt for blood tests to monitor methylene blue levels in the body and adjust dosages accordingly under medical guidance.
5. **Avoiding Self-Medication:** Always discuss with a healthcare professional before starting methylene blue treatment, especially if you're already taking other medications or have underlying health conditions.

While methylene blue can be an incredible tool in our health toolkit, it demands respect when it comes to dosing. It's about finding that sweet spot where benefits outshine risks without venturing into unfamiliar territory without proper knowledge or guidance.

I am continually encouraged by the strides we're making in understanding alternative therapies like methylene blue in supporting mitochondrial function. By staying informed and cautious about dosages, we can safely explore its revolutionary potential together. Remember, these guidelines are a starting point—your optimal dose may require adjustments based on personal needs and professional advice.

Combination With Other Treatments

We all know that our bodies have little powerhouses called mitochondria. They're crucial for generating energy that we need for everything—from moving our muscles to keeping our brains sharp. However, when these powerhouses start failing, it leads to many diseases. Here's where methylene blue comes in. It's like giving these mitochondria a much-needed boost, enabling them to work efficiently.

Now, imagine pairing methylene blue with other therapies—this tandem approach might just be revolutionary in combating diseases. Let me share some fascinating combinations of treatments involving methylene blue.

One interesting partner is hyperbaric oxygen therapy (HBOT). You might have heard of this therapy being used for divers or healing tissue damage after injury. When combined with methylene blue, HBOT seems even more promising. It floods your system with pure oxygen under pressure, increasing overall oxygenation in tissues and organs. When cells have more oxygen, they're better at using energy. The synergy between HBOT and methylene blue amplifies their individual benefits—like putting two good friends in the same room and watching them support each other's strengths.

Let's also talk about light therapy—a form of treatment where specific wavelengths of light are used to treat certain conditions. When methylene blue is used alongside red or near-infrared light therapy, it's believed that the photoreceptors in our cells absorb this light and function more efficiently. The roles of both partners complement one another beautifully: while light therapy enhances cellular energy levels, methylene blue helps maintain efficient energy production.

For those dealing with mental health challenges like depression or anxiety, combining methylene blue with cognitive-behavioral therapy (CBT) or medication could yield promising outcomes. Why would this work? While CBT helps rewire thought patterns and medications manage neurotransmitter levels, methylene blue targets another essential layer by improving cellular respiration in the brain, allowing treatments to work more effectively.

In addition to these combination possibilities, many experts are exploring the dual use of supplements like CoQ10 or NAD+ precursors alongside methylene blue. These supplements naturally boost mitochondrial function on their own and when paired with methylene blue, patients may experience enhanced energy levels and an improved sense of well-being.

These combinations warrant further exploration through clinical trials; they're still in early phases but experimental data seems very encouraging indeed. That's not to say these are magical solutions—in healthcare nothing ever is—but the possibility that such combinations can help mitigate suffering should fill us all with hope.

COMBINATION THERAPY	POTENTIAL BENEFITS
Methylene Blue + Hyperbaric Oxygen	Enhanced oxygenation; improved mitochondrial efficiency
Methylene Blue + Light Therapy	Increased cellular energy output; improved cell performance
Methylene Blue + CBT/Medications	Enhanced cognitive benefits; improved mental health outcomes
Methylene Blue + Supplements	Boosted mitochondrial function; enhanced physical vitality

Long-Term Use

Methylene Blue has the ability to remain effective over extended periods. When we think about using any treatment long-term, several crucial factors come into play, including efficacy, safety, and possible side effects. Based on current research and long-standing studies, Methylene Blue demonstrates remarkable traits in all these areas.

Studies suggest that Methylene Blue maintains its support for cellular health even with prolonged use. Many participants report sustained improvements in energy levels, cognitive function, and overall well-being. Its role in preserving mitochondrial function appears not only to stabilize but to enhance over months and years of utilization.

When it comes to safety, progressive research reassures us about its profile during extended use. While no treatment is without potential side effects, Methylene Blue is generally well-tolerated by the majority of users when used appropriately. Of course, it's always essential to monitor personal responses and consult healthcare professionals for tailored guidance.

An aspect often brought up in discussions is the long-term impact on mental health. Intriguingly, some studies highlight its antidepressant-like effects might persist or even amplify over time. It's surmised that Methylene Blue may fortify brain health through enhancing mitochondrial efficiency and neuro-protective properties.

EFFECT	INITIAL (1-3 MONTHS)	EXTENDED (6-12 MONTHS)	LONG-TERM (+12 MONTHS)
Energy Levels	Improved	Consistently High	Very High Sustainment
Cognitive Function	Noticeable Enhancement	Stable Enhancement	Adaptive Sharpening

| Mental Health | Uplifted Mood | Signs of Stability | Increasing Resilience |
| *Overall Well-being* | Heightened Awareness | Balanced Improvement | Maintained Vitality |

This chart reflects general trends noted by researchers including myself. However, individual experiences may vary greatly due to unique biological factors. A frequently asked question revolves around the practicality of using Methylene Blue daily beyond the one-year mark. Given its benefits, many find it complementing their lifestyle choices seamlessly—like maintaining a regimen or routine that supports their health goals.

As part of understanding Methylene Blue's place in life-long wellness strategies, more observational studies will be invaluable. The more data we collect over time from diverse user groups across varying health conditions, the better we understand how optimally integrate Methylene Blue into holistic wellness plans without compromising other aspects of health management such as diet or exercise routines.

Personalized Treatment Plans

Personalized treatment is about recognizing that each of us is unique. Our bodies react differently to medications based on genetics, health history, lifestyle, and even environment. This is why a one-size-fits-all approach can often fall short in effectively managing many conditions. Personalized treatment acknowledges this diversity and adapts accordingly.

Methylene blue has shown incredible potential across an array of medical conditions due to its capacity to enhance mitochondrial function. However, even as effective it is broadly, customizing its application could significantly boost its impact. Imagine two patients presenting similar symptoms but having different underlying biological conditions; they might benefit from variations in dosage or combination therapies that precisely address their unique health situations.

To create a personalized methylene blue treatment plan, the first step often involves comprehensive diagnostics. By using advanced genetic testing and biomarker analysis, we can gain valuable insights into a patient's specific biological makeup. This allows us to predict how they might respond to methylene blue and identify the optimal dose needed for maximum benefit while minimizing adverse effects.

Let's say we have Alice and Ben, two hypothetical patients suffering from similar symptoms associated with mitochondrial dysfunction. Genetic analysis shows that Alice may metabolize medications quicker than Ben due to certain enzyme variations. This means Alice might require a slightly higher dose of methylene blue to achieve therapeutic effects compared to Ben. On the other hand, Ben may have a genetic disposition that makes him more susceptible to potential side effects at standard doses. Therefore, starting him off at a lower dose before gradually increasing it could be more suitable.

Additionally, tracking biomarkers specific to mitochondrial health over time during treatment can provide feedback on how well the therapy is working and if adjustments need to be made. Personalized plans don't just stop at adjusting dosages either: they also involve considering other lifestyle factors that might support or hinder treatment efficacy.

For instance, incorporating dietary recommendations that enhance mitochondrial function alongside methylene blue can potentially amplify results. This aligns with emerging research suggesting that diet plays a crucial role in how our bodies respond to treatments by affecting cellular energy production pathways.

Below is a simplified table representing key factors considered in personalizing methylene blue treatments:

FACTOR	CONSIDERATION
Genetic Profile	Affects drug metabolism rate
Biomarker Levels	Determines baseline mitochondrial health
Lifestyle Habits	Diet and exercise impact cellular energy balance
Environmental Exposure	Potential influence on oxidative stress levels

Incorporating these elements into each treatment plan isn't just about efficiency—it's about ensuring care that's as safe and effective as possible for every individual under our guidance. It's important we keep abreast of ongoing studies exploring how best methylene blue treatments can be fine-tuned based on personal health profiles—this knowledge base only continues expanding!

By embracing personalization in our methodologies today despite challenges inherent in broad application shifts (like cost or accessibility), we're laying groundwork not just for mitigating disease but ultimately fostering holistic long-term well-being tomorrow—one uniquely tailored pathway at time!

BOOK 3
METHYLENE BLUE FOR DISEASE TREATMENT

CHAPTER 5
DISEASES TREATED BY METHYLENE BLUE

Neurodegenerative Diseases

Neurodegenerative diseases, as many of you might know, include familiar names such as Alzheimer's, Parkinson's, and Huntington's disease. These are conditions defined by the progressive degeneration or death of nerve cells. This process can lead to problems with movement (ataxia) or mental functioning (dementia).

Methylene Blue's track record with neurodegenerative conditions primarily revolves around its ability to support mitochondrial activity—the powerhouses in our cells that are critical for energy production. In simpler terms, think of it as providing a boost to your cell's energy factories, which might be flagging due to illness.

In Alzheimer's disease, one of the key challenges is the accumulation of protein clumps called amyloid plaques and tau tangles. These disrupt normal cellular operations and lead to neuron death. Methylene blue is believed to have properties that may help prevent or reduce these buildups. What's fascinating is that by enhancing mitochondrial function, methylene blue could potentially arrest or even reverse some of the cognitive declines associated with Alzheimer's.

Then there's Parkinson's disease, where dopamine-producing neurons in a part of the brain called the substantia nigra begin to deteriorate. This causes the motor symptoms most people associate with Parkinson's — tremors, rigidity, and slowness of movement. The exact mechanisms are still under research, but current findings suggest that methylene blue may help by stabilizing neuronal energy supply and reducing oxidative stress, another villain that's often up to no good in these diseases.

Huntington's disease is yet another realm where methylene blue might shine. It's a genetic disorder that affects muscle coordination and leads to cognitive decline and psychiatric problems. Given its hereditary nature, identifying effective treatments has been particularly challenging. However, early-stage research indicates that methylene blue might aid in maintaining neuronal integrity longer than previously possible.

While promising results have emerged from studies and trials so far, we're still on this exploratory journey together — myself along with many dedicated colleagues worldwide who are testing this compound's limits and potentials. Our collective efforts will indeed shed more light on how effectively we can harness methylene blue's neurological benefits without significant side effects.

DISEASE	ROLE OF METHYLENE BLUE
Alzheimer's	Reducing plaques & tangles
Parkinson's	Antioxidant action against free radicals
Huntington's	Potential stabilization of mitochondrial function

It's important during this exploration process that we express both enthusiasm and caution—current studies show promise but are in no way conclusive yet. The molecular details around how MB operates are still being investigated but what keeps us inspired is its potential backed by initial findings from both cellular models and some animal studies.

As we progress further into understanding these diseases and refining treatments like those involving Methylene Blue, continuous research will be essential. Staying informed empowers us: whether you're specifically dealing with these diseases or simply across the broader spectrum interested in health-related science developments.

Metabolic Disorders

Metabolic disorders are a diverse group of conditions that affect the body's ability to properly turn food into energy. This process involves complex chemical reactions, and when something goes awry, it can lead to a range of health issues. Interestingly, Methylene Blue has shown promise in tackling some of these disorders.

A key player in energy production is the mitochondrion—the powerhouse of the cell. In a variety of metabolic disorders, mitochondrial dysfunction is a common feature. This is where Methylene Blue steps in with its unique ability to enhance mitochondrial performance.

Let's focus on one notable disorder—Chronic Fatigue Syndrome (CFS). This condition leaves individuals feeling utterly exhausted with minimal effort, often accompanied by muscle pain and concentration difficulties. The underlying cause isn't fully understood, but researchers suspect mitochondrial dysfunction plays a crucial role.

Here's where Methylene Blue provides hope. By improving electron transport within mitochondria, it helps cells produce more ATP—the primary energy currency of our bodies. Many people with CFS who have tried Methylene Blue report noticeable improvements in their energy levels and overall functioning.

Another application is with Metabolic Syndrome—a cluster of conditions including increased blood pressure, high blood sugar levels, excess body fat around the waist, and abnormal cholesterol levels. Even though lifestyle changes like diet and exercise are critical here, Methylene Blue might offer additional support.

In laboratory studies, Methylene Blue has been seen to improve insulin sensitivity—a major issue for those dealing with Metabolic Syndrome or Type 2 Diabetes. By helping cells respond better to insulin, it aids in maintaining blood sugar levels within a healthy range.

Mitochondrial dysfunction is known to contribute significantly to insulin resistance. With its ability to enhance mitochondrial efficiency, Methylene Blue provides a promising adjunctive therapy alongside conventional treatments.

Now let's look at Phenylketonuria (PKU), a rare inherited disorder where one's body can't break down an amino acid called phenylalanine. If untreated, phenylalanine can build up and lead to brain damage and other severe health problems.

While adhering to a strict diet low in phenylalanine remains the cornerstone for managing PKU, research suggests that Methylene Blue might offer complementary benefits. It supports cellular metabolism and reduces oxidative stress—a condition linked closely with PKU and many other metabolic disorders.

METABOLIC DISORDER	ROLE OF METHYLENE BLUE
Chronic Fatigue Syndrome	Enhances mitochondrial function for better energy production
Metabolic Syndrome	Improves insulin sensitivity; supports glucose regulation
Phenylketonuria (PKU)	Reduces oxidative stress; supports cellular metabolism

This table illustrates how Methylene Blue could potentially support individuals suffering from various metabolic disorders through different mechanisms tied to cellular energy production and reducing stress at the cellular level.

Cardiovascular Health

Methylene blue has been shown to help with cardiovascular diseases by acting as an antioxidant within our blood vessels. By reducing oxidative stress, it protects the lining of these vessels, which is crucial because oxidative damage can lead to conditions like hypertension and atherosclerosis. These are fancy terms for high blood pressure and hardened arteries, respectively—both of which significantly increase the risk of heart attack and stroke.

But what does acting as an antioxidant actually mean? Think of oxidation as rusting — not on metal but in our bodies. This "*rust*" can damage cells over time. By preventing this oxidative stress, methylene blue helps maintain smoother operations within the body's cardiovascular system.

A key factor in cardiovascular health is the function of endothelial cells that line blood vessels. Healthy endothelial cells promote proper dilation and contraction of blood vessels, ensuring good blood flow. Methylene blue helps improve the function of these endothelial cells, keeping our blood vessels flexible and responsive.

Now, let's discuss how methylene blue affects blood pressure—an essential aspect of heart health. It seems to lower blood pressure moderately by improving nitric oxide availability. Nitric oxide is a molecule that relaxes blood vessels, allowing blood to flow more freely and reducing the pressure in those vessels. Think of it like widening a narrow road to reduce traffic congestion.

Another vital area where methylene blue has shown promise is protecting healthy heart muscle cells while inhibiting unwanted cell growth—a delicate balance important for maintaining strong heart function. This becomes especially crucial in conditions like cardiac hypertrophy, where the heart muscle thickens excessively due to increased workload or stress.

In addition to cellular protection, methylene blue also influenced energy production in cardiac cells through enhanced mitochondrial function (without diving deep into its workings here). Healthier mitochondria result in more efficient energy use by heart cells during each beat—a critical factor for optimal cardiac performance.

The immune response involved in cardiac inflammation also interplays with methylene blue's therapeutic effects on the cardiovascular system. Conditions like myocarditis involve inflammation of the heart muscle, often resulting from viral infections or other causes. Here, methylene blue acts beneficially by modulating this inflammation so as not to overwhelm delicate heart tissues.

ASPECT	ROLE OF METHYLENE BLUE
Antioxidant Action	Reduces oxidative stress; protects vessel walls
Endothelial Function	Improves vessel dilation/contraction; maintains healthy flow
Blood Pressure	Lowers via enhanced nitric oxide availability; reduces vessel strain
Cellular Protection	Preserves heart muscle cells; prevents unwarranted cell growth
Energy Production	Enhances mitochondrial activity; optimizes cardiac energy usage
Inflammation Modulation	Manages inflammatory response; prevents excessive inflammation

It's crucial to underline that while existing research highlights these promising effects, direct clinical application still demands cautious consideration and consultation with healthcare professionals. What works well in laboratory settings may differ from individual responses depending on other variables such as current health status or concurrent treatments one might be undergoing.

Immune System Support

Your immune system is your body's defense network, aglow with soldiers that fight off invaders like bacteria, viruses, and other harmful agents. Over time, due to stress, infection, or other factors, our immune defenses can falter. Methylene Blue steps in as an assistive agent for this massive army—the immune system. It acts like a guardian ensuring that cells function optimally. One of its key roles includes reducing oxidative stress. Oxidative stress is like rust on metal—it decays the cell structures and hampers their function. Methylene Blue helps to protect these cells by neutralizing oxidative agents.

Think of it this way: these protective measures allow the battalions inside you (B cells and T cells) to operate smoothly without wasting energy dealing with the molecular equivalent of pot holes on a road. If we visit another avenue—antimicrobial properties—Methylene Blue has shown promise here too. To put it in perspective, consider how sunlight sanitizes surfaces by breaking bacteria down; similarly, Methylene Blue can enhance cellular protection mechanisms against microbes.

It was interesting to find applications point toward improving the effectiveness of existing treatments. In some instances where traditional antibiotics struggle, this blue dye offers additional support by enhancing cellular uptake and improving bacterial eradication rates. That means in simpler terms: it helps your immune system be a little more effective at tackling those nastier bugs without needing to up the dose on prescriptions.

Next up is energy production as an immune booster; without adequate energy production within our cells (thanks to our dear mitochondria), our immune response could feel more like sluggish defeat than energetic readiness. So *how does Methylene Blue come into play?*

Imagine mitochondria as the powerhouse managers—they transform nutrients we consume into usable energy forms (ATP). Methylene Blue supports energy production efficiency by allowing these powerhouses to produce ATP more effectively during cellular distress or disease impacts ensuring that when there's an all-hands-on-deck situation inside due to invading pathogens - A.K.A germs - power surges instead of browning out! Energy reserves mean more power for your immunity team!

ASPECT	ROLE OF METHYLENE BLUE
Oxidative Stress	Decrease (20% reduction reported)
Antimicrobial Effectiveness	Up to 2x improvement when combined treatment
Energy Production	Steady preservation/increase (significant boost in ATP levels)*

*Note: The precise impact may vary based on individual health conditions and existing levels of mitochondrial dysfunction.

We must acknowledge realistic boundaries too—while promising studies hydrate curiosity pools abundantly—more diving regarding long-term usage outcomes reinforce conclusions needed today globally still remains undisclosed data.

Mental Health Conditions

Depression is one condition wherein methylene blue shows considerable promise. Consider it as a potential backdrop rather than a one-size-fits-all solution. Depression affects millions globally, often manifesting as persistent sadness, lack of interest in activities once enjoyed, and even profound physical ailments. Traditional treatments include antidepressants and therapy; however, not everyone finds relief through these means. That's where methylene blue comes in, potentially offering a new ray of hope.

The way methylene blue works with the brain is quite fascinating. It enhances the electron transport chain within our cells' powerhouses, the mitochondria, improving their efficiency. By doing so, it can potentially elevate mood by aiding better cellular energy production—a fundamental aspect when considering conditions like depression, where sluggish cellular activity is often observed.

Beyond depression, anxiety disorders are another area under exploration. These disorders can be exceptionally crippling, resulting in constant worry or fear that seems uncontrollable. Emerging studies suggest that methylene blue might help modulate neurotransmitters involved in mood regulation such as serotonin and dopamine.

MENTAL HEALTH CONDITION	ROLE OF METHYLENE BLUE
Depression	Enhances mitochondrial function, potentially boosting mood

Anxiety Disorders	Modulates neurotransmitters like serotonin and dopamine
Bipolar Disorder	May stabilize mood swings through improved cellular function
Cognitive Impairment	Supports cognitive function by optimizing brain energy metabolism

While research is still ongoing, the bipolar disorder community has begun discussing methylene blue as well. The stability of mood swings in bipolar disorder patients has shown potential improvement with this treatment. Often known for extreme highs and lows, any tool that could guide individuals toward equilibrium is worth investigating.

Cognitive impairment related to diseases such as Alzheimer's or simply age-associated cognitive decline also adds another dimension to methylene blue studies. There's an exciting possibility that it can enhance overall brain energy metabolism, potentially staving off cognitive deficits or slowing down their progression.

I must remind you that though compelling evidence continues to surface, the administration of methylene blue for mental health purposes should always be under professional guidance. Understanding precise dosages and potential interactions with other medications is crucial for ensuring safety and efficacy.

Lastly, imagine your brain cells as tiny power plants—when they don't work optimally due to mitochondrial dysfunctions or resultant chemical imbalances associated with various psychiatric conditions—it could lead you into those darker alleyways of mental health struggles. With its ability to invigorate these cells' energy output perhaps derived from years spent understanding nuances of medicine—it's clear why there's excitement surrounding this humble yet versatile compound's emergence onto mental health radars worldwide.

CHAPTER 6
REVOLUTIONARY TREATMENT PROTOCOLS

Dosage for Various Diseases

When it comes to exploring alternative treatments for diseases, especially those linked to mitochondrial dysfunction, finding the right dosage is crucial. Remember that individual variations exist, so it's always prudent to consult a healthcare professional in any treatment regimen. The effectiveness of Methylene Blue can vary depending on the condition being treated. The idea is to provide just enough to stimulate beneficial effects without causing any adverse reactions.

Let's start by looking at neurodegenerative diseases such as Alzheimer's and Parkinson's. Research suggests that a lower dose could be beneficial here. Typically, doses ranging from 0.5 mg/kg to 4 mg/kg of body weight per day are considered safe and effective. What does this mean? If you're weighing around 70 kg (about 154 pounds), your daily intake should steer between 35 mg and 280 mg.

For mood-related disorders like depression or anxiety, Methylene Blue might be used at doses similar to or slightly lower than those used for neurodegenerative diseases. Frequently, a range of 0.5 mg/kg to 2 mg/kg daily is recommended as these doses tend to show promise in lifting mood and enhancing cognitive function without overwhelming systemic effects.

Interesting findings have emerged indicating that Methylene Blue can serve as an antimicrobial agent under certain circumstances due to its ability to produce a high amount of reactive oxygen species upon exposure to light. In these cases, dosage could play a critical role. Typically, an effective dose falls within the broader range we discussed earlier; however, for acute infections, some therapies utilize a slightly higher concentration under guided supervision.

With cancer treatment protocols in mind, things get more intricate. While research is ongoing and often studied in vitro or animal models, similar ranges have been observed effective—starting low and adjusting as necessary depending on observed tolerance and response. Again, staying within the parameters of around 1 mg/kg seems optimal pending further long-term studies.

DISEASE TYPE	RECOMMENDED DOSAGE
Neurodegenerative	0.5 - 4 mg/kg per day
Mood Disorders	0.5 - 2 mg/kg per day
Infectious Diseases	Adjusted case-by-case
Cancer Approaches	Variable; seek guidance

Remember: more isn't necessarily better with interventions like these. Half-life considerations where Methylene Blue can linger in the system up to several hours support once-daily or divided dose approaches depending on one's specific needs. While promising advancements are being made day by day—as researchers and practitioners gather more substantial evidence—it remains integral that we balance vigilance in application with openness toward emerging insights on optimal strategies moving ahead.

Combination Therapies

You might wonder, what exactly is a combination therapy? It's like teaming up a group of superheroes to defeat a common enemy. By using two or more treatments together, we can create a synergy that enhances the effects of each individual option, making them more potent in addressing diseases.

In the revolutionary treatments, Methylene Blue has shown incredible promise. Pairing it with other therapies can enhance its potential even further. Let's explore some exciting combination protocols that are being studied and show serious potential.

1. Methylene Blue and Antioxidants: A Power-Packed Duo

Imagine Methylene Blue as an artist carefully restoring an old painting. It works on improving cellular function by enhancing mitochondrial activity. Now, picture adding antioxidants to this mix—they're like the protective coating that prevents future damage. When we combine these two treatments, they help mitigate oxidative stress while boosting overall cell health.

2. Methylene Blue with Hyperbaric Oxygen Therapy

Hyperbaric Oxygen Therapy (HBOT) involves breathing pure oxygen in a pressurized room or chamber. It increases oxygen delivery to tissues and promotes healing—not unlike an oxygen supercharge for your cells! When combined with Methylene Blue, HBOT enhances oxygen availability even more within the mitochondria, amplifying energy production and providing remarkable results across several conditions.

3. Working Alongside Nutritional Supplements: A Holistic Approach

Nutritional supplements like Coenzyme Q10 (CoQ10) or L-carnitine play a significant role in mitochondrial health. Suppose we introduce Methylene Blue into this holistic treatment plan—it's akin to giving these nutrients an extra boost! This partnership supports better energy metabolism and fosters cellular vitality.

COMBINATION THERAPY	BENEFITS
MB + Antioxidants	Reduces oxidative stress; boosts cell health
MB + HBOT	Enhances oxygen availability; improves energy production

| MB + Nutritional Supplements | Supports energy metabolism; promotes cellular vitality |

4. Pairing with Light Therapy: Enhancing the Cellular Symphony

Specific wavelengths of light have been shown to stimulate cellular processes significantly when used correctly. By incorporating light therapy with Methylene Blue, it's as if we're fine-tuning a symphony—each part perfectly enhancing the other—resulting in optimized cellular functions which promote healing and regeneration.

5. Utilizing Exercise Protocols Alongside Treatments

Exercise is undoubtedly essential for overall well-being; now consider pairing moderate physical activity with our beloved Methylene Blue regimen! Physical movement aids mitochondrial function naturally—it encourages them to produce more ATP (energy currency), leading it into harmony with Methylene Blue's actions boosts overall treatment effectiveness.

Combination therapies pave pathways towards innovation within alternative medicine practices globally since they hold great potential against otherwise stubborn health challenges such as neurodegenerative diseases or chronic fatigue syndrome-like symptoms!

Treatment Timelines

When considering any new protocol, it's vital to develop a comprehensive timeline—one that not only outlines the daily and weekly application of a treatment but also considers how treatments might evolve based on progress and any potential side effects. In my research, I've found that this structured approach helps maximize therapeutic benefits while minimizing risks.

One important aspect to consider is the initial phase of introducing a new treatment. This phase typically involves starting with a low dose or minimal intervention to assess tolerance and compatibility with the individual's existing condition. Depending on the treatment's complexity and the patient's response, this phase may last anywhere from a few days to several weeks. During this time, close monitoring of one's reaction to the treatment is recommended.

After establishing tolerance, we move into what I'd call the "*ramp-up phase*." This phase involves gradually increasing the treatment's intensity or dosage, allowing the body to acclimate without overwhelming it. The length of this phase can widely vary but often spans from two weeks to several months. The key here is incremental adjustment—fine-tuning the protocol according to the patient's unique response patterns.

It's critical during these stages to engage in active communication with healthcare providers to ensure safety and address any concerns promptly. This partnership helps in adapting treatment pacing based on individual needs rather than following a rigid, one-size-fits-all timeline.

For some conditions or patients, entering a "maintenance phase" marks an important transition in their healing journey. In this stage, patients continue an effective dose or routine that sustains achieved benefits without seeking further escalation. The duration of maintenance can vary immensely; some individuals may maintain certain protocols for life, while others might need adjustments seasonally or as their health evolves.

Understanding when and how to taper off—or even discontinue—a particular protocol is another critical aspect of these timelines. Tapering requires careful consideration to prevent rebound effects or loss of health gains previously accomplished. For example, slowly reducing treatment over weeks (or sometimes months) can be essential for maintaining balance within the body.

It is also crucial not to overlook periodic reassessment stages within your timeline—a moment when evaluating how far one has come versus where they need to go next occurs. These reassessments allow for necessary adjustments based on new insights into personal health data and advancements in broader medical research findings.

PHASE	DURATION	PURPOSE
Initial Phase	Days to Weeks	Assess tolerance; establish baseline
Ramp-up Phase	Weeks to Months	Gradually increase dose/intensity
Maintenance	Varies widely	Sustain benefits without further escalation
Tapering	Weeks to Months	Prevent rebound; safely reduce/discontinue
Reassessment	Throughout timeline	Regularly evaluate progress and adjust as needed

This structured approach allows us to break down what can often feel overwhelming into manageable steps, ensuring we address each aspect of treatment thoughtfully and methodically. By following these phases, we can adapt the timeline to fit individual needs and responses, making sure that the protocols remain as effective as possible.

Although the framework provides a clear guide, it is essential to remain open to adjustments. Health conditions are dynamic, and what works at one stage might need transformation at another. The beauty of this approach lies in its adaptability—it encourages tailoring treatments while acknowledging individual variability.

Moreover, having a structured timeline can reduce anxiety for both patients and healthcare providers by clarifying expected progress and potential pivots if necessary. This clarity facilitates more targeted interventions and timely adjustments, potentially leading to better health outcomes.

Case Studies and Patient Stories

Case Study 1: Alzheimer's Disease and Cognitive Decline

Our first case focuses on a patient we'll call Linda, a 68-year-old woman who had been experiencing progressive cognitive decline over several years. Her family noticed her increasing forgetfulness and episodes of confusion. After being diagnosed with early-stage Alzheimer's, they sought options beyond conventional treatments.

With Linda's condition, we aimed to address mitochondrial dysfunction as a potential underlying factor in her cognitive issues. It was essential to devise a protocol that might improve her quality of life and potentially slow the progression of the disease.

Treatment Protocol:

1. *Supplement Regimen:* Linda was introduced to a regimen of supplements known for supporting mitochondrial function, including CoQ10 and alpha-lipoic acid.
2. *Dietary Adjustments:* Her diet was optimized to enhance mitochondrial efficiency, emphasizing foods rich in antioxidants and omega-3 fatty acids.
3. *Methylene Blue Therapy:* We employed low-dose Methylene Blue as part of her daily protocol, known from previous discussions for its role in enhancing cellular respiration and energy production.

Over the course of six months, Linda experienced noticeable improvements. Her episodes of confusion diminished significantly. We observed an overall stabilization in her cognitive abilities, which was quite promising given the typical trajectory of Alzheimer's symptoms.

ASSESSMENT	BASELINE	AFTER 6 MONTHS
Memory recall tests	Poor	Improved
Confusion frequency	Frequent	Rare
Quality of life score	Low-Med	Medium

Case Study 2: Chronic Fatigue Syndrome (CFS)

The second case involved a gentleman, David, aged 45, bedridden by relentless fatigue. Diagnosed with Chronic Fatigue Syndrome (CFS), he had struggled for years with limited success from conventional treatments. David's journey led him to us in search of something more radical. Given CFS's complex nature—often involving several body systems—we decided to focus on energizing his mitochondria to counteract his fatigue.

Treatment Protocol:

1. **Energy Boosting Supplements:** A combination of NAD+ boosters and riboflavin was introduced to enhance energy production.
2. **Physical Activity Routine:** A gentle exercise program tailored to his energy levels aimed at gradually increasing his stamina without causing the classic post-exertional malaise.
3. **Methylene Blue Administration:** Integrating Methylene Blue proved pivotal, as it supports improved efficiency in cellular processes essential for energy.

The transformation over eight months was profound. David reported a gradual increase in energy levels and achieved consistent progress. He managed basic activities that were previously daunting and reclaimed a sense of normalcy.

ACTIVITY LEVEL	INITIAL STATUS	STATUS AFTER 8 MONTHS
Morning routine	Bedridden	Independently mobile
Exercise tolerance	Very low	Moderately active
Overall stamina	Drained	Noticeably improved

These cases highlight the vitality that can be restored through alternative protocols targeting mitochondrial health. While traditional methods remain crucial in clinical practice, such revolutionary approaches offer additional avenues for patients desiring comprehensive treatments.

It is exciting to witness firsthand how these protocols yield tangible benefits, affirming the potential lying within innovative sciences like these.

Patient Story 1: Arnold's Journey to Renewal

Arnold was a 56-year-old teacher who had been experiencing persistent fatigue and brain fog. These symptoms had steadily worsened, affecting his ability to perform daily tasks and maintain his quality of life. Traditional treatments offered little relief and prompted Arnold to explore alternative options.

When Arnold first learned about the treatment protocol involving Methylene Blue, he was intrigued but cautious. After a comprehensive discussion with his healthcare provider, he decided to give it a try. The protocol was tailored specifically for him, focusing on gradual incorporation into his routine.

Within weeks of starting the protocol, Arnold reported noticeable improvements. His energy levels began to soar, and the fog that clouded his thoughts started to clear. This progress wasn't just anecdotal; it was supported by tangible metrics from regular doctor visits.

Dramatic Improvements Observed:

>   *Before:* Severe fatigue, frequent brain fog
>   *After:* Enhanced energy levels, clarity in thought processes

Arnold's work life also improved as he regained his vigor and enthusiasm for teaching. He noted how these improvements allowed him not only to work effectively but also to engage in activities that he once loved but had abandoned due to his exhaustion.

Patient Story 2: Susan's Path to Health

Susan was a 42-year-old graphic designer who battled with chronic migraines and an overwhelming sense of lethargy. After exhausting conventional methods without success, Susan turned her attention to revolutionary treatment protocols.

Her journey with the new protocol was another testament to its potential. Like David, Susan noticed enhancements in her condition fairly early on. Her migraines became less frequent, providing her with much-needed relief from constant discomfort.

A fascinating aspect of Susan's case was the improvement in her creative output—the very essence of her profession. Susan mentioned that her newfound health allowed her creativity to flourish once more, leading to both professional satisfaction and personal joy.

Notable Outcomes for Susan:

>   Before: Regular migraines, low energy
>   After: Reduced migraine occurrences, heightened energy levels

These personal accounts highlight the transformative power of integrating Methylene Blue into treatment plans for complex conditions associated with mitochondrial dysfunction. These stories belong not just to David or Susan but resonate with anyone seeking hope through newly opened doors in healthcare innovation—an innovation everyone deserves access to when traditional routes may falter.

Monitoring Health Improvements

When we're trying out any treatment, especially those that address mitochondrial dysfunction — complex issues that underlie many diseases — it's crucial we have clear markers of improvement. You'd be surprised how small changes can signal big improvements over time.

The Role of Biomarkers

Think of these as footprints left behind when something changes in your body — they tell us where you've been and where you're heading with your health journey. If the treatments are working, these footprints will lead us towards health and away from disease. Identifying the right biomarkers is crucial because they help us target our therapies better and adjust them as needed. Some common biomarkers include:

1. **Energy Levels:** People often notice changes in their overall energy levels. An increase in sustained energy throughout the day is a good sign that your mitochondria are functioning better.
2. **Inflammation Markers:** Tests can show if inflammation in the body decreases with treatment. Lower inflammation often correlates with improved mitochondrial function.
3. **Oxidative Stress Markers:** These measure the balance between free radicals and antioxidants in your body, providing information about cellular health.

While some people might have access to advanced medical resources, I advocate for simple tools accessible to everyone. Here are some easy ways anyone can keep tabs on their progress:

1. **Journaling:** Keeping a daily log of symptoms, mood, energy levels, sleep quality, and exercise can reveal patterns over time.
2. **Wearables:** Fitness trackers or smartwatches can be great for monitoring heart rate variability, sleep patterns, and even activities like steps or cycling.
3. **Apps:** There are plenty of apps designed to track various health metrics which make monitoring easier than ever before.

While these tools provide insights on a daily basis, remember they're not absolute measures but great for showing trends over time.

Below is a simple chart example that might help visualize how one could record some common observations during this treatment protocol:

WEEK	ENERGY LEVEL (1-10)	SLEEP QUALITY (1-10)	INFLAMMATION SCORE	ADDITIONAL NOTES
1	4	5	High	Noticed fatigue
2	5	6	Moderate	Slight increase in alertness
3	6	7	Moderate	Energy spikes during midday
4	7	8	Low	Consistent physical activities unexhausted

The key here isn't just the raw numbers — it's about seeing where they go over several weeks or months.

By consistently tracking various aspects of your well-being with these markers and tools, we can adjust treatments effectively. Remember that these improvements may not always come quickly; sometimes they're subtle shifts over time. But with patience and dedication to monitoring these signs, it's possible to guide health outcomes positively.

BOOK 4
PROTOCOLS FOR WELL-BEING

CHAPTER 7
REVOLUTIONARY TREATMENT PROTOCOLS

Personalized Treatment Plans

When it comes to health, the days of the one-size-fits-all approach are fading fast. Instead, there's a growing emphasis on personalized medicine—something that really resonates with me as a medical researcher focused on mitochondrial health and alternative treatments.

Imagine walking into a doctor's office and instead of receiving conventional advice that broadly targets your symptoms, you leave with a treatment plan created just for you. This is the power of personalized treatment—your unique biology guides your path to health. We take into account everything from your genetic makeup to your lifestyle, environment, and even your gut microbiome.

Why tailor treatments? Mitigating disease is not just about stopping symptoms but nurturing overall well-being—and there's no better way than personalizing a plan that fits like a glove. The starting point often involves comprehensive testing. Genetic testing can unearth biological pathways related to diseases. Meanwhile, epigenetic testing provides insights into how lifestyle and environment may affect gene expression. This combination gives us a clearer picture so we can arm ourselves with the right tools.

After gathering this plethora of information, the next step is crafting the personalized treatment protocol. Here's where things get creative and truly customized. One of the keystones of this process is functional medicine—a field dedicated to identifying and treating root causes—not just symptoms. Functional medicine practitioners focus on individualized care using interventions like dietary modifications, lifestyle changes, and novel therapies that are perfect fits for specific biological needs.

For example, someone might benefit from an altered diet—to add or eliminate certain foods—to improve gut health or inflammatory conditions which are hallmarks of mitochondrial dysfunction. In addition to dietary guidance, supplements can play a crucial role in personalized protocols. These may include vitamins, amino acids, probiotics or antioxidants—all selected based on individual necessity rather than general advice.

To illustrate the scope of personalization in wellness plans, consider the following simplified chart outlining common tests/assessments used in personalizing treatments:

TESTS/ASSESSMENTS	PURPOSE
Genetic Testing	Identifies predisposition to various health conditions
Metabolic Panel	Highlights current metabolic functions
Microbiome Analysis	Reveals gut health and impacts nutritional absorption
Hormonal Profile	Unveils imbalances impacting physical/emotional well-being
Food Sensitivity Testing	Helps identify potential triggers causing inflammation

With this information at hand—armed with knowledge about your body's intricate workings—we aim not just to treat but to empower you toward greater vitality.

Beyond tests and supplements lies another crucial aspect: lifestyle interventions adapted specifically for you—whether they involve stress reduction methods like meditation or yoga tailored according your daily stresses—or customized exercise regimens designed around current fitness levels paired effectively against preventing disease progression while promoting mitochondrial well-being.

Individual feedback loops create yet another layer of customization within personalized treatment plans. This dynamic process means your treatment evolves as you do, adjusting to changes in your health and lifestyle for the most effective results. Picture this: regular check-ins with healthcare providers to assess how treatments are working for you. It's like having a personal health coach who ensures your plan stays relevant, altering it whenever necessary to keep pace with your life.

Let's say you've begun a stress reduction routine that includes yoga and meditation, but after a few weeks, you notice it's not quite doing the trick for your stress levels. A personalized plan allows for adjustments—perhaps incorporating different mindfulness techniques or evening walks if they suit you better.

Moreover, personalized treatment protocols benefit from technology. Smartphones and wearables can track everything from sleep patterns to heart rates, offering real-time data that provides insights into what's working and what's not. This is immediate feedback at its finest, where information gathered can shape the next step of your wellness journey.

Connecting all these dots results in a treatment plan that acknowledges the complexity of human health—not by simplifying it into one-size-fits-all solutions but by embracing it. Personalized approaches recognize that what works wonders for one person might not be as effective for another, honoring our diversity in health responses and needs.

For those committed to maintaining mitochondrial well-being specifically, adopting such tailored treatment strategies could redefine their approach to health entirely. Instead of quick fixes or temporary solutions, what's offered is enduring wellness informed by their biology and lived experiences.

Dosage Guidelines for General Well-Being

When thinking about using methylene blue for general well-being, it's essential to consider how this compound can affect you personally. The beauty of well-being treatment protocols lies in their adaptability. There isn't just one way to apply them; rather, there's a spectrum of possibilities tailored to individual needs.

A critical factor in using methylene blue effectively is understanding the right dosage. This isn't about throwing caution to the wind but carefully considering your body's responses and consulting with healthcare professionals when needed. The general approach involves starting with a conservative dose and observing how your body responds. Over time, and with professional guidance, adjustments help you hit that sweet spot where you feel more lively and centered.

Here's an overview of typical dosage guidelines for general well-being:

DOSE CATEGORY	ESTIMATED AMOUNT	FREQUENCY	OBSERVATIONS
Initial Low Dose	0.5 mg per kg body weight	Once daily	Ideal for newcomers to assess tolerance
Moderate Dose	1 mg per kg body weight	1-2 times daily	For those who demonstrate good initial response
Personalized Optimal Dose	Varies based on individual reactions	As advised by health provider	Tailored for personal goals

It's crucial to mention that everyone's response can differ due to various factors like lifestyle, diet, and even psychological disposition. Therefore, listening to your body is key. Let's discuss everyday scenarios where methylene blue might fit into an individual's routine for general well-being:

1. **Enhanced Mood and Energy:** Users often report feeling more energetic and positive after incorporating initial doses into their morning routines. This boost can be complementary to other lifestyle habits like regular exercise and a balanced diet.
2. **Cognitive Clarity:** Another common benefit people notice when taking methylene blue is an increase in mental sharpness. It's as though a fog lifts, making it easier to concentrate on tasks at hand. Many use a moderate dose in their morning routine to support clarity throughout the day, finding it beneficial for work or study sessions. The experience can be similar to when you have that perfect cup of coffee—an instant spark to get going without the jittery side effects.
3. **Stress Management:** Balancing work, family, and personal commitments can be overwhelming, leaving one feeling drained and anxious. Methylene blue users often report a sense of calm that facilitates better stress management. Implementing it in the evening, perhaps after dinner, might help unwind and alleviate the stress accumulated over the day, supporting a restful night's sleep.
4. **Physical Endurance and Recovery:** Engaging in regular physical activities is fundamental for well-being. Some people notice improved stamina and quicker recovery times when incorporating methylene blue into their wellness regimen. It might pair well with your post-workout shake or supplement stack. People often benefit from starting with a low dose immediately after exercise sessions to aid muscle recovery.

5. **Immune Support:** While methylene blue isn't a replacement for vaccines or other medical interventions, users suggest it could provide adjunctive support for overall immune function. Adhering to the conservative initial doses may align with personal health goals during flu season or times of increased physical demands.
6. **Holistic Support:** Incorporating methylene blue into your routine isn't just about addressing isolated aspects of health but viewing your body as an interconnected system. Through careful dosage personalization—which often entails liaising with healthcare providers—a holistic approach enables individuals to optimize overall health.

Below is a simplified example of how you might track doses along with subjective observations:

DAY	DOSE	TIME TAKEN	EFFECTS/NOTES
1	0.5 mg/kg	Morning	Slight mood uplift
2	0.5 mg/kg	Morning	More energy
3	0.5 mg/kg	Evening	Better sleep quality

This table serves as a framework for monitoring initial doses and observing how different times of the day influence outcomes. Adjustments should only happen once there's a consistent pattern of how you feel at certain doses over several days—discuss any changes with your doctor before proceeding.

Long-Term Methylene Blue Usage

Despite its humble origins as a dye, researchers are continuously discovering its versatile capabilities. Using this compound over extended periods requires careful consideration of both physiological impacts and psychological perceptions. We know methylene blue has a unique ability to cross the blood-brain barrier. This attribute makes it particularly effective in addressing neurological aspects of well-being when used long-term. From improving cognitive function to moderating mood disorders, it's like having an all-in-one supplement keyed directly to nervous system optimization. I believe its utility lies in the consistency of small doses rather than large episodic uses, thereby integrating it into daily life much like traditional vitamin supplements.

One area where my research shows promise is mental clarity. The mental fog some experience due to high-stress lifestyles can potentially be mitigated by consistent methylene blue usage. Users have reported enhanced focus and greater clarity during tasks that require prolonged attention—think of it as fine-tuning your brain's operating system for peak efficiency.

This effect extends to emotional stability too. Chronic stress is rampant today, and managing it is key to long-term health. Here's where methylene blue shines—users have observed a reduction in anxiety symptoms and improved mood regulation over time.

Beyond neurological benefits, methylene blue seems to offer support to bodily functions at a cellular level. Studies point out its role in energy production improvement by acting semi-antioxidant—reducing oxidative stress significantly when used continuously. Over time, individuals have noticed improvements in their physical stamina and a greater sense of vitality.

When contemplating its integration into lifestyle routines, it's crucial to account for dietary factors that might influence absorption rates and efficacy. Maintaining optimal hydration levels and ensuring nutrient-rich meals can significantly amplify methylene blue's benefits, creating a synergistic environment for promoting health.

However exciting these benefits might sound, I cannot overstate the importance of being aware of potential drawbacks associated with long-term use. Periodic assessment by healthcare professionals familiar with your individual needs should accompany extended use since changes at the cellular level could manifest differently across biochemical compositions.

One potential risk includes methemoglobinemia—a condition where oxygen delivery through blood could be impeded—but this is generally rare with low-dose regimens. Monitoring standardized blood work regularly can prove beneficial in catching any anomalies early on.

Furthermore, documenting personal reactions over extended periods through journaling or apps can help in tailoring regimens to manage side effects effectively if they arise unexpectedly. Here's a simple chart representing the potential benefits identified versus documented risks over long-term usage:

POTENTIAL BENEFITS	POTENTIAL RISKS
Improved cognitive function	Methemoglobinemia
Reduced oxidative stress	Possible mild nausea
Enhanced emotional stability	Skin discoloration (rare)
Increased physical vitality	Headaches (occasional)

I hope this chart helps illustrate that while there are numerous advantages to prolonged methylene blue use, keeping informed about the subtle risks becomes imperative during regular adoption into daily protocols.

Monitoring Progress and Adjustments

Embarking on any health journey or treatment protocol is akin to setting out on an adventure; there will be discoveries, challenges, and adjustments along the way. When we introduce methylene blue into the equation, its effects may begin to manifest subtly but significantly. Each person is unique, with their own biology and responses, which makes it paramount to monitor progress closely and adjust treatments accordingly.

Monitoring one's response to treatment serves as both a compass and a map. It helps to guide you through the effectiveness of the interventions you're undertaking. *How do we go about it in a manner that's both comprehensive and uncomplicated?* Let me take you through some straightforward strategies that I have found useful.

Keeping a daily log can be incredibly insightful. A simple notebook or digital app where you jot down how you're feeling each day acts as a personal progress journal. Note things like energy levels, cognitive function, mood changes, sleep patterns, and any physical symptoms. You'll find that over time, patterns begin to emerge. These patterns are pivotal in determining if and how well the treatment is working for you.

DAY	ENERGY LEVEL (1-10)	MOOD (1-10)	SLEEP QUALITY (POOR/FAIR/GOOD)	NOTES

1	5	6	Fair	Felt sluggish in the afternoon
2	6	7	Good	Woke up feeling refreshed
3	7	6	Fair	Had trouble focusing

This table can help provide a visual representation of your progress over time. Noticing a consistent rise in energy levels or improved sleep quality could confirm that your therapy is on the right track.

Regular check-ins with your healthcare provider are essential in this process. They can offer insights based on professional experience and probably notice trends that might escape your self-monitoring efforts. Together, you can make informed decisions when it comes to any necessary adjustments in dosage or technique.

Occasionally, adjustments are imperative for optimal results. Your logs may show stagnant progress or even regressive trends necessitating tweaks in your approach. Adjustments might involve recalibrating dosages postpartum or finding alternative schedules that better fit your lifestyle.

As with all treatments, the goal is not simply remediation but enhancement of overall well-being. Consider incorporating supportive lifestyle changes such as balanced nutrition, moderate exercise, adequate sleep hygiene, and stress management techniques. These not only aid methylene blue's potential benefits but contribute holistically to one's health.

It's natural to encounter roadblocks during any protocol adaptation phase—plateaus where improvements seem at a standstill or days when setbacks threaten motivation. This is when patience and persistence are key allies—the understanding that healing isn't linear; it's dynamic.

Lastly—but crucially—be kind to yourself throughout this journey. Celebrate small victories as indicators of growth rather than solely seeking monumental shifts overnight. This adaptive approach recognizes our adaptive nature and the unique paths each of us undertakes towards improved well-being. It's about being present and attentive to our body's feedback, using these cues to shape our interventions proactively. Our ability to adjust and refine treatments over time is a celebration of how personalized medicine can be empowering.

Consider this journey as an exploration of what works best for you, not just in terms of physical health but also emotional and mental rejuvenation. By engaging in this process, you're actively participating in your wellness narrative—paving your own path to enhance vitality and resilience through mindful adjustments and dedicated monitoring.

Moreover, sharing experiences with others who are also exploring methylene blue treatments can be immensely supportive. It builds a community of collective learning where insights are exchanged, helping everyone refine their approaches. Remember, you're not alone in this endeavor; many have embarked on similar journeys striving for well-being.

Always remain honest with yourself regarding how you feel day-to-day. This honesty is crucial for accurately gauging progress and knowing when it's time for change. The ultimate aim is crafting a protocol that seamlessly integrates with your life's rhythm—maximizing benefits while supporting harmony in your daily routines.

Integrating Methylene Blue with Other Supplements

When we talk about revolutionary treatment protocols, integrating methylene blue with other supplements is a potential catalyst for enhancing well-being. This combination can offer holistic health benefits by addressing various aspects of physiological functions.

One supplement I've found particularly interesting when combined with methylene blue is Coenzyme Q10 (CoQ10). Many of you might know CoQ10 as a key player in energy production within our cells. By pairing it with methylene blue, we're looking at a duet that can harmonize cellular respiration and energy synthesis. This combo may help propel mitochondrial function to new heights, providing an energy boost that can enhance physical and cognitive performance.

Another noteworthy partner is N-acetylcysteine (NAC), which acts as a precursor to glutathione, one of our body's most powerful antioxidants. When methylene blue's antioxidant properties meet NAC's ability to replenish intracellular levels of glutathione, the protective framework within our cells is significantly reinforced. Together, they work diligently to mitigate oxidative stress—a common culprit behind chronic diseases and aging.

Let's not overlook Vitamin B12 either. Many methylating agents have shown promise in enhancing mood and cognitive abilities. Methylene blue combined with B12 can fortify neurological health by supporting nerve cell integrity and neurotransmitter function. It's a combination that many find beneficial in improving mental clarity and focus.

Consider also the role of Magnesium. This mineral aids numerous biochemical reactions in the body and is known for its calming effects on the nervous system. When integrated with methylene blue, magnesium may support metabolic efficiency and muscle relaxation, potentially reducing the stress load on both mind and body.

SUPPLEMENT	POTENTIAL SYNERGISTIC EFFECTS WITH METHYLENE BLUE
Coenzyme Q10 (CoQ10)	Enhances energy production; boosts mitochondrial efficiency
N-acetylcysteine (NAC)	Reduces oxidative stress; replenishes vital antioxidant stores
Vitamin B12	Improves neurological health; supports nerve cell function
Magnesium	Promotes metabolic balance; provides calming effects

Understanding these interactions is crucial for creating personalized protocols aimed at well-being enhancement through supplementation. However, it's essential to approach this intelligently—monitoring individual responses and tweaking treatment plans accordingly.

With any protocol involving supplements, especially potent ones like methylene blue, starting low and going slow cannot be emphasized enough. This allows us to monitor our responses carefully and adjust dosages sensibly. Pairing your observations with regular consultations with healthcare providers ensures safety

Starting with low doses of methylene blue and gradually increasing as tolerated is the general approach I recommend. This allows for careful observation of how your body responds to the supplement mixture, ensuring that any adverse reactions are caught early and managed appropriately. Consulting with a healthcare provider familiar with these types of supplements can also provide additional guidance tailored to individual needs.

It's important to pay attention to how you feel during this process. Are you experiencing an increase in energy levels, improved clarity of thought, or perhaps a deeper sense of relaxation? These could be signs that the combination is benefiting your mitochondrial function and overall well-being. On the other hand, if you're feeling more fatigued or experiencing any unusual symptoms, it would be wise to reassess your protocol or seek professional advice.

We should remember, too, that these supplements should complement a healthy lifestyle. Proper nutrition, regular exercise, and sufficient sleep are all fundamental to maintaining high-functioning mitochondria. When combined with the right supplements, including methylene blue and its counterparts like CoQ10, NAC, Vitamin B12, and Magnesium, we create a formidable plan for enhancing our well-being.

Regular check-ins with yourself—and possibly your healthcare provider—can help you determine whether adjustments are needed. Personalized supplementation protocols are as much about fine-tuning as they are about foundational knowledge and initial planning.

CHAPTER 8
INTEGRATING METHYLENE BLUE FOR WELL-BEING

Daily Routines

If you are new to using Methylene Blue, it is essential to start with a low dosage and gradually increase as necessary. It helps to record the effects on your body and mind to find the right amount that benefits you personally. Remember, each individual's needs may vary, so listen to what your body is telling you.

Establishing a routine with Methylene Blue can be straightforward if incorporated mindfully. Perhaps the most logical way to begin is by considering when in your day you might benefit the most from its energy-boosting properties. Some people prefer to take it in the morning with their breakfast. This timing can provide an early surge of energy that helps kick-start their day, enhancing clarity and focus.

On the other hand, there are those who feel they have a significant slump post-lunch, where productivity could be bolstered by a small dose of Methylene Blue. For them, integrating it into an afternoon ritual—perhaps taken alongside a cup of herbal tea—can reinvigorate their mental faculties for the remainder of the day.

Consistency is key when adding any new supplement or compound into your regimen. Whatever time you choose for ingestion, try to stick with it consistently so that your body builds an intuitive response over time. Much like any health-related practice, such as mindfulness or even brushing your teeth, regularity breeds familiarity—and effectiveness.

While considering timing, it's good to pair Methylene Blue with periods of mental activity when possible due to its cognitive-enhancing capabilities. Utilizing short windows of focused work or study sessions can amplify its effectivity.

For those curious about direct application methods for physical ailments like skin issues or localized discomforts, creating a topical solution might be beneficial after consulting with healthcare professionals on safety practices. Direct usage varies substantially from oral intake; hence expertise guidance is paramount here.

TIME	ACTIVITY	POTENTIAL BENEFIT
Morning	Breakfast schedule	Initial energy boost; heightened focus
Post-Lunch	With midday relaxation/mental preparation	Combats afternoon slump; renewed clarity
Pre-Study	Before intensive cognitive activities	Enhanced mental acuity

Remember always to hydrate adequately when taking Methylene Blue, as staying well-hydrated aids in balancing its effects—an aspect easily overlooked but critical in maintaining overall well-being. Always keep track of how you're feeling over intervals by noting any patterns or changes observed over weeks; this real-time feedback will assist in calibrating its role within your daily practices effectively.

And for those who are constantly on the go, integrating Methylene Blue into a travel routine can prove invaluable. Imagine preparing for a long-haul flight or a busy day of meetings—keeping a small vial handy can provide a necessary lift when feeling jet-lagged or mentally drained. However, always remember to follow airline regulations and pack it safely.

Many who have successfully incorporated Methylene Blue into their routine note the importance of creating a simple tracking system. They find that keeping a small journal or using an app to jot down the time, dosage, and any notable effects throughout the day gives essential insights into how it influences their mood and energy levels.

A useful addition to your routine might be setting alarms or reminders. Just like taking medications or vitamins, setting electronic reminders ensures doses aren't missed and become part of your daily habit seamlessly. Don't hesitate to discuss your experiences with Methylene Blue with like-minded communities or forums if available. Sharing insights can offer new perspectives and recommendations that you might not have considered on your own. It's about building a supportive network where experiences enrich collective knowledge.

As we explore Methylene Blue's integration into daily routines, it's clear that it's about finding what works best for you and weaving it into your life's rhythm comfortably and reliably. Remember, patience is fundamental while you adapt and refine this new part of your well-being routine.

Nutrition And Supplementation

In recent years, the exploration of alternative and supportive approaches to health and well-being has led to renewed interest in methylene blue. Though originally synthesized in the late 19th century, its application extends to various domains of wellness today.

Owing to modern agriculture and food processing, it's often argued that essential nutrients found in our daily diet aren't as abundant—or bioavailable—as they once were. This is where methylene blue enters the conversation, offering an intriguing option thanks to its potential cellular benefits.

Methylene blue is perhaps most celebrated for its supportive role in combating mitochondrial dysfunction, a condition linked with various diseases and age-related decline. By aiding the mitochondria—the powerhouses of our cells—methylene blue helps optimize energy production, thereby potentially boosting vigor and vitality.

Integrating methylene blue doesn't mean upending your entire dietary routine but rather enhancing it thoughtfully. Many adhere to this supplementation through oral intake as part of their morning or evening regimes, similar to how one might add vitamins or minerals.

1. **Dosing:** Typical doses might range from 0.5mg to 4mg per kilogram of body weight, although it's crucial to consult healthcare professionals before initiating any new supplement.
2. **Combination with Other Nutrients:** Pairing methylene blue with antioxidants such as vitamin C could further bolster its effectiveness by combating oxidative stress—essentially cellular rust that can accelerate aging and disrupt normal cell function.
3. **Form:** Choosing the right form is vital; pharmaceutical-grade methylene blue ensures purity and safety compared to industrial-grade alternatives which might contain impurities unsuitable for human consumption.

Through a nutritional lens, methylene blue holds promising anti-inflammatory qualities which could aid those grappling with chronic inflammation—a common thread in many modern ailments.

To illustrate, consider Jane, who integrates methylene blue into her daily nutrition plan alongside improved hydration and balanced meals—rich in leafy greens like spinach known for their mitochondrial support vitamins like A and K. Over several months, she reports increased clarity in thought and physical endurance—small changes but noteworthy steps towards enhanced quality of life.

As part of a broader approach, meals enriched with omega-3 fatty acids (found in salmon or chia seeds) complement the action of methylene blue beautifully; both support brain health while promoting cellular resilience. Here's a simple table showcasing how you might structure a day's meals incorporating these principles:

MEAL	COMPONENTS
Breakfast	Oatmeal with chia seeds & blueberries
Snack	Mixed nuts (almonds & walnuts), herbal tea
Lunch	Spinach & quinoa salad with grilled salmon
Snack	Apple slices with almond butter
Dinner	Grilled chicken, roasted vegetables

The intrigue surrounding methylene blue isn't without scientific backing. Studies suggest it may protect nerve cells against injury from free radicals while stabilizing mood over prolonged use—a testament to its wide-ranging impact when thoughtfully integrated into one's nutritional habits.

However, promising these prospects seem, caution is paramount. Individual responses can vary significantly; hence starting at lower dosages while monitoring one's personal experience becomes key. Always engage with healthcare practitioners when contemplating new additions or changes surrounding supplements like methylene.

Preventative Health Strategies

In recent years, a growing interest in preventative health strategies has emerged, and with good reason. As the saying goes, an ounce of prevention is worth a pound of cure. By taking proactive steps, we can fortify our bodies against potential ailments and promote overall well-being. One intriguing addition to this wellness toolkit is methylene blue, a compound with a long history of use and a promising future in healthcare.

Methylene blue is making waves in the world of health for its potential protective properties. Originally used as a dye and later as a treatment for malaria, it is now being explored for its ability to support our body's resilience against various diseases. As part of a preventive strategy, integrating methylene blue into your routine could provide significant benefits without waiting for issues to arise.

Methylene blue stands out because it can cross the blood-brain barrier, reaching areas that many compounds cannot. Its ability to reach different parts of our body means it can potentially aid in more than just one specific area. It helps by increasing the efficiency of cellular respiration—the process by which our cells produce energy from the food we eat. This improved energy production might play a crucial role in maintaining cell health and reducing the risk of developing chronic conditions.

Moreover, methylene blue has antioxidants properties. Antioxidants are substances that help reduce damage from oxidative stress—a process that can contribute to aging and various diseases. By combatting these oxidative stresses, methylene blue may act as a safeguard for our cells.

Using methylene blue as part of a preventive strategy doesn't mean overhauling your entire lifestyle. Instead, it's about incorporating it thoughtfully into daily practices. One area where methylene blue shows great promise is cognitive health. As we age or face daily stressors, the brain's performance can suffer. Methylene blue's ability to enhance mitochondrial function might help protect brain cells from degenerative changes. While it's not a miracle solution, it could be an ally in maintaining clarity and focus.

Another preventative application lies in supporting our immune system's robustness. Methylene blue might improve cellular activity that fights infections and pathogens by enhancing cellular energy production and antioxidant defense mechanisms.

POTENTIAL BENEFIT	HOW METHYLENE BLUE HELPS
Cognitive Health	Enhances energy production in brain cells
Immune Function	Boosts cellular defense mechanisms
Cellular Longevity	Provides antioxidant support

When considering adding methylene blue into your wellness regimen, several practical points are worth noting:

1. **Dosage:** Start low and slow—the key is finding the right balance without overwhelming your body.
2. **Safety First:** Consultation with healthcare professionals is essential to ensure safety, especially if you are taking other medications or have underlying health issues.
3. **Observation:** Keep track of how your body responds; everyone's experience can vary.

As with any supplementation approach, personalized guidance based on individual needs and conditions is crucial. This helps ensure that every step taken aligns with personal health goals without unintended consequences.

The prospect of integrating methylene blue into preventive health strategies represents a shift towards proactive wellness management. While research continues to unravel its full potential, current insights offer exciting possibilities for enhancing human well-being from within.

Exercise And Lifestyle Factors

Exercise isn't just about keeping the waistline in check or building muscle. It's a remarkable part of enhancing our energy levels and overall health. Regular physical activity naturally boosts our mood, as it triggers the release of feel-good hormones called endorphins. But did you know that combining this with Methylene Blue can amplify these benefits?

Methylene Blue works as a powerful aid in optimizing energy production at the cellular level. It acts like a helper in your cells, making sure your little energy factories are running smoothly and efficiently. When paired with exercise, it provides an additional boost to cellular energy, improving both performance and recovery.

Imagine this as fueling up your car before embarking on a long drive. With a full tank (thanks to exercise), and an engine tuned to perfection (via Methylene Blue), you're all set for an optimal journey.

When you think about your day-to-day activities, aim for at least 150 minutes of moderate aerobic exercise each week combined with strength-training exercises twice per week. This basic guideline can transform everything from mood to metabolism. When you incorporate Methylene Blue into this routine, you are effectively 'double-dipping' into wellness. Think of Methylene Blue like the secret sauce for amplifying workout effects:

1. **Enhanced Endurance:** Whether you're running a marathon or just taking a brisk walk, you'll likely find that stamina improves.
2. **Quick Recovery:** Post-exercise fatigue reduces considerably, meaning less soreness and quicker readiness for your next workout.
3. **Greater Focus:** Exercise also helps clear our minds, but with Methylene Blue, increased mental clarity becomes evident much faster.

At this point, these combinations might sound too good to be true but trust me—they're completely backed by science.

Creating an optimal lifestyle goes beyond achieving personal bests at the gym; it's about maintaining balance within daily activities. Here's how you could potentially integrate these elements:

1. **Mindful Movement:** Dedicate time each day for activities that don't feel like exercise—dance around your living room or bike ride along scenic routes.
2. **Social Connections:** Engage in group activities wherever possible—hiking clubs or sports teams foster connections while increasing motivation to remain active.
3. **Rest is Essential:** Proper rest is crucial! It's nature's way of ensuring your body repairs itself properly—enhanced even further with supportive aids like Methylene Blue.

Integrating these adjustments takes time, so always approach changes gradually rather than aplenty at once.

DAY	ACTIVITY	DOSE
Monday	Walking 30 mins	MB supplement
Wednesday	Strength Training	MB supplement
Friday	Yoga or Tai Chi	MB supplement
Saturday	Group activity (hike)	MB supplement

The proposed schedule encourages variation while keeping consistent doses aligned throughout the week—not necessarily every single day—ensuring sufficient rest time amid active days.

Stress Management

Stress is something we all face in our daily lives. Whether it's work pressures, family responsibilities, or unexpected life events, stress can feel overwhelming. It's essential to have effective strategies to manage it. One intriguing approach is the integration of methylene blue, a compound that some researchers are exploring for its potential benefits in stress management.

Methylene blue has a long history of use, primarily known as a dye and an antiseptic. However, recent investigations highlight its role in enhancing cellular energy production. This property might make it a promising ally in dealing with stress. *But how exactly?*

When we're stressed, our bodies react by producing hormones like cortisol and adrenaline. While these hormones are useful in short bursts—like running away from danger—they aren't great when they flood our system continuously. Over time, high stress levels can affect mental clarity, mood stability, and overall health.

Methylene blue potential lies in how it can boost energy at a cellular level without adding more physical energy demands on the body. It seems to optimize how cells use oxygen and produce energy. This increased efficiency could help mitigate the fatigue and brain fog often associated with chronic stress.

Imagine your body as a factory: during stressful times, requests (or tasks) for productivity shoot up dramatically—but sometimes the machines (your body's cells) can't keep up due to resource limitations or inefficiencies in production lines (energy pathways). Methylene blue's role would be like upgrading these machines so that they perform better under pressure without breaking down.

Here's how you might think about incorporating methylene blue into your stress management toolkit safely:

1. **Start Small:** Like any new supplement, it's crucial to begin with a low dose and observe your body's response. Consult with a healthcare professional before starting any new supplement regimen.
2. **Consistency is Key:** Regularity can enhance potential benefits. Think about incorporating it gradually into your schedule rather than as an immediate fix during peak stress moments.
3. **Combine Efforts:** Remember that methylene blue isn't a miracle cure-all. For best results, integrate it alongside other holistic practices such as mindfulness meditation or yoga—which directly manage stress—and healthy lifestyle choices already discussed in previous sections.
4. **Monitor Effects:** Keep track of any changes you notice once you start using methylene blue regularly—like your energy levels throughout the day or your ability to handle challenging situations calmly.

To make this easier to digest, let's look at how integrating methylene blue could fit within a basic weekly plan:

DAY	ACTIVITY
MON	Begin morning with deep-breathing exercises
TUE	Add 0.5 mg/kg methylene blue after breakfast
WED	15-minute walk during lunch break
THU	Mindfulness meditation for 10 minutes before bed
FRI	Review week's stressors; practice gratitude journaling
SAT	Evaluate mood changes; adjust methylene dosage if needed

| SUN | Reflect on overall wellness and plan next week |

This table offers a simple strategy where the integration of methylene blue complements other tried-and-tested stress-reducing habits. When considering any new intervention such as this one for managing stress effectively—it's all about balance. We want improved well-being without creating dependencies or overlooking fundamental lifestyle factors that contribute equally to our health.

Consider this holistic approach as an opportunity to create harmony rather than relying solely on one solution. Yes, methylene blue can be a valuable asset in our stress-management toolkit, but it's most effective when used alongside other positive habits. The key is to maintain a rounded approach that includes not just supplements, but also practices that nurture your mind and body in different ways.

BOOK 5
PREVENTATIVE AND LIFESTYLE CARE

CHAPTER 9
PREVENTATIVE HEALTH STRATEGIES

Importance Of Preventative Care

Many people only visit their doctor when something is wrong or they're experiencing symptoms, but *what if we could avoid these problems by taking steps to prevent them in the first place?* That's where preventative health strategies come into play. By focusing on prevention, we can maintain our wellbeing over the long term and avoid serious health issues before they arise.

Preventative care means anticipating and managing potential health problems early on before they develop into more serious conditions. Think of it like maintaining a car. Regular oil changes and tune-ups can keep your vehicle running smoothly and prevent major breakdowns. Similarly, by incorporating preventative measures now, we may sidestep major health concerns down the road.

One key role of preventative care is identifying risk factors associated with common illnesses. Risk factors might include lifestyle choices like poor diet and lack of exercise or genetic predispositions that you might be aware of due to family history. By understanding these patterns, you can take proactive actions that reduce your risk. For instance, if you're predisposed to cardiovascular issues, monitoring blood pressure and cholesterol levels regularly can be vital.

Immunization is another essential part of prevention. Vaccines help protect against infectious diseases by preparing your immune system to fend off viruses and bacteria before they become a problem. Ensuring that immunizations are up to date can save you from potentially severe health complications later in life.

Stress management is another component worth considering in preventative care strategies. Stress is often called a silent killer because it contributes to various health problems such as heart disease, diabetes, and mental health issues like depression or anxiety. Learning techniques to manage stress effectively—be it through meditation, yoga, or hobbies—can have profound effects on both mental and physical health.

Protecting ourselves from harm shouldn't only be about tackling what's inside our bodies; it's about considering how external risks affect us too. Safety measures such as wearing seat belts in cars or helmets when biking are forms of daily prevention that protect against unforeseen accidents.

Preventative care also includes fostering good communication with healthcare professionals. Regular visits to doctors help spot potential issues early on while encouraging an open dialogue about any changes in your body or concerns you may have.

The benefits of adopting a preventative health strategy are vast. Not only does it potentially extend longevity, but it also saves money in the grand scheme of healthcare costs by reducing hospital visits and minimizing the need for expensive medical treatments resulting from unchecked diseases.

PREVENTATIVE MEASURES	BENEFITS
Regular Exercise	Improves overall fitness; reduces disease risk
Balanced Diet	Supports immune function; controls weight
Vaccinations	Protects against infectious diseases
Stress Management	Enhances mental wellbeing; reduces illness
Screening Tests	Early detection of potential issues

Incorporating these easy yet effective strategies into everyday life isn't just about living longer; it's about improving quality at every stage along the way. Investing time into prevention today creates a healthier tomorrow.

The importance of preventative care lies fundamentally in its power to secure not just mere survival but a thriving existence teeming with vitality and robustness through each phase of life's journey. Prevention may not be treated with urgency since it deals with potentialities rather than current certainties—but its impact resonates deeply across years to come.

Building A Healthy Lifestyle Foundation

Taking charge of your health can seem overwhelming. However, adopting preventative health strategies is one of the most effective ways to ensure long-term wellness and build a robust foundation for a healthy lifestyle. By focusing on aspects that influence our daily lives, we can take significant steps toward preventing diseases and enjoying a vibrant life.

1. **Importance of Sleep and Rest**: A key pillar in creating a healthy lifestyle is prioritizing sleep and rest. Quality sleep is not just about feeling refreshed the next day; it plays a crucial role in cell repair, muscle growth, and immune function. Consistent sleep patterns help regulate hormones related to hunger and stress, minimizing the risk of conditions such as obesity and depression.

Consider setting a regular bedtime to align with your natural circadian rhythm. Ideally, adults should aim for 7-9 hours of sleep per night. Creating a calming bedtime routine — perhaps by shutting down electronic devices an hour before bed or indulging in a warm bath — can signal to your body that it's time to relax.

2. **Mental Health Awareness**: Mental health is intricately connected to physical well-being, forming an integral part of preventative health strategies. Proactively managing stress through mindfulness practices such as meditation or yoga can enhance emotional resilience. These practices help lower stress hormones while increasing serotonin levels, which contribute to happiness and calmness.

Don't hesitate to reach out for support if needed. Talking with friends, family, or mental health professionals can offer fresh perspectives and encourage emotional healing.

3. **Hydration: An Often Overlooked Component**: Staying hydrated is often overlooked but essential for maintaining bodily functions. Water aids digestion, nutrient absorption, and toxin elimination from the body. Even slight dehydration can lead to fatigue, headaches, and impaired concentration.

Strive to drink at least 8 cups (64 ounces) of water daily — more if you're physically active or live in hot climates. Be mindful of sugary drinks or excessive caffeine; they can lead to dehydration over time.

4. **Cultivating Social Connections**: Human beings are inherently social creatures, so nurturing social connections is vital for our health. Positive relationships provide emotional support that buffers against stress and has been associated with longer life expectancy.

Make an effort to strengthen relationships by spending quality time with loved ones or engaging in community activities that interest you. Surrounding yourself with supportive individuals fosters self-esteem and reduces feelings of loneliness or isolation.

5. **Embracing Physical Activity Beyond Exercise**: It's crucial not only to focus on structured workouts but also on increasing overall daily movement — whether it's choosing stairs over elevators or taking regular walks during breaks at work. Prolonged periods of inactivity are detrimental; therefore, incorporating small changes like standing desks or active commuting helps counteract their effects.

See below for an easy-to-follow chart illustrating ways to incorporate more movement into your day:

DAILY MOVEMENT IDEAS	APPROXIMATE CALORIES BURNED/HOUR*
Walking (3 mph)	210
Gardening	250
Biking (leisurely pace)	280
House Cleaning	180
Dancing	330

*NOTE: *Caloric burn estimates vary based on individual's weight and intensity level.*

By integrating preventive strategies such as focusing on sleep quality, mental well-being, proper hydration habits alongside fostering social connections — all complemented by increased physical activity -- you'll establish sturdy foundations conducive towards living healthier lives collectively!

Routine Health Screenings

One essential aspect of ensuring long-term health is preventative healthcare, specifically through routine health screenings. Imagine taking your car for a maintenance check to catch minor issues before they become major problems—routine health screenings serve a similar role for your body. These screenings are like a roadmap to detecting diseases early on when they are most treatable and manageable. They help identify risks and health conditions early, potentially saving lives and improving your overall quality of life.

Routine health screenings are medical tests or examinations aimed at checking for signs of disease before symptoms appear. The frequency and types of screening tests recommended can vary based on age, gender, family history, lifestyle choices, and other risk factors. For example, while women might be advised to get regular mammograms to screen for breast cancer, men might have prostate exams as they age.

Let's break it down further by age group:

1. **Young Adults (Ages 18-39):**

Blood Pressure Measurements: High blood pressure can go unnoticed without visible symptoms. Regular checks help prevent future heart diseases.

Cholesterol Levels: Starting in your 20s, get your cholesterol checked every 4-6 years.

2. **Middle-Aged Adults (Ages 40-59):**

Type 2 Diabetes Screening: With the onset of middle age and possible weight gain or lifestyle changes, screening becomes important.

Eye Exams: To catch signs of glaucoma or vision changes early.

3. **Older Adults (Ages 60 and Older):**

Bone Density Test: Screening for osteoporosis becomes crucial as bones naturally weaken with age.

Colonoscopy: To screen for colorectal cancer from ages 50 onwards (or earlier depending on risk factors).

Alongside these targeted screenings based on age and gender-specific needs, there are universal checks that everyone should consider regularly—skin checks for abnormal moles or growths that could indicate skin cancer, dental exams to maintain oral health which is linked to heart health, and hearing tests to catch potential issues before they impact your lifestyle.

But why stop at just listing tests? Let's look at the benefits these screenings offer:

1. **Early Detection and Treatment:** Many serious conditions like cancers or heart diseases can develop quietly without showing symptoms until advanced stages. Early detection via screenings means diseases can be treated more effectively.

2. **Peace of Mind:** Regular check-ups provide reassurance about your health status. Knowing you're doing what you can to stay healthy offers significant peace of mind.

3. **Lifestyle Adjustments:** Screenings often reveal lifestyle-induced conditions like high cholesterol or hypertension allowing individuals to make proactive changes in their diet or exercise routines.

Remember that while the thought of medical appointments may not top anyone's list of favorite activities, they should be viewed as empowering steps towards taking charge of your own health.

Nutritional Strategies for Disease Prevention

It's not just about reacting to illnesses but taking proactive steps to stop them in their tracks, or better yet, ensuring they never come knocking at all. Interestingly, nutrition plays a pivotal role in this preventive landscape. As we move forward in unpacking these strategies, let's discuss some insightful yet simple methods to harness the power of food for disease prevention.

Foods rich in nutrients contribute significantly to our health and well-being and can reduce the risk of various chronic diseases. By including a wide array of fruits and vegetables in our diet, we're essentially giving our bodies the antioxidants they need to fight off harmful oxidative stress. This stress is a major player in the development of conditions like heart disease and cancer.

1. **Fiber:** Found abundantly in whole grains, fruits, and vegetables — fiber is incredibly important for maintaining digestive health. It lowers cholesterol levels and aids in controlling blood sugar levels, thus reducing the risk of type 2 diabetes.
2. **Omega-3 Fatty Acids:** These healthy fats, present in foods like fish (think salmon or mackerel), flaxseeds, and walnuts, have been shown to reduce inflammation. Chronic inflammation is linked with various diseases such as arthritis and even Alzheimer's disease.
3. **Vitamins and Minerals:** Essential vitamins like C and D, along with minerals such as zinc and magnesium, support everything from immune function to bone health. Vitamin C-rich foods like citrus fruits aid collagen synthesis for skin strength and elasticity.

Providing regular nourishment to your body isn't merely about choice but necessity in preventing illness. An interesting approach to consider is the Mediterranean diet — known for its emphasis on plant-based foods along with healthy fats from olive oil and fish. Studies suggest that this diet significantly lowers cardiovascular risk factors compared to typical Western diets laden with processed meats and refined sugars.

Now let's look at a simple table illustrating how switching certain "*less beneficial*" choices for more nutrient-rich alternatives can impact your overall health:

INSTEAD OF...	TRY...
Sugary snacks	Fresh fruit or nuts
Soda	Herbal tea or infused water
White bread	Whole-grain bread
Processed meats	Lean poultry or legumes

By making these minor tweaks to your eating habits, you're not just feeding yourself; you're also nurturing your long-term vitality. What's crucial here is balance and consistency. While it's tempting to focus on individual "*superfoods*," true dietary success lies more broadly in variety — consuming a colorful mix of plants guarantees a range of protective nutrients.

Furthermore, hydration should never be underestimated as part of nutritional strategy for disease prevention. Water is fundamental for bodily functions — from temperature regulation to joint lubrication — making it integral to sustaining life itself.

Adopting these nutrition strategies doesn't require revolutionary changes in one's lifestyle; it's about making conscious, incremental changes that collectively lead to significant health benefits. Remember, taking small steps every day can yield impressive long-term results.

Role Of Environmental Factors in Health

Think of your environment as everything that surrounds you every day—it's the air you breathe, the food you eat, the water you drink, and even the lights and sounds that fill your world. Understanding these elements can empower you to make choices that support your well-being.

The Air We Breathe

Clean air is vital to our health. Unfortunately, air pollution is everywhere and can harm our respiratory health. Pollutants such as smog, smoke, and dust can get into our lungs and bloodstream, leading to serious conditions like asthma or other respiratory issues. To protect yourself, try to stay informed about air quality in your area—many cities have apps or websites that can tell you the daily air quality index.

On a practical level, indoor air quality is just as important as outdoor. Some simple things you can do include using air purifiers at home, ensuring good ventilation when cooking or painting, and having houseplants like spider plants or peace lilies to help clean the air naturally.

The Water We Drink

Access to clean water is crucial since it's used for drinking, cooking, and cleaning. Contaminants in water such as lead or bacteria can pose serious health risks. It's essential to be aware of your local water quality reports and consider using filters if needed. At home, boil your water if you're uncertain about its safety or use certified filtration systems that meet standards for removing specific impurities.

Food Quality and Safety

Our food environment includes not just what we eat but also where it comes from and how it's produced. Eating foods that are less processed and rich in natural ingredients lowers exposure to harmful chemicals often found in preservatives or artificial additives.

Shopping at farmers' markets or choosing organic produce when possible helps ensure you're consuming fewer pesticides. Moreover, being mindful of food labeling allows for better choices regarding additives and potential allergens.

Noise Pollution

Have you ever thought about noise affecting your health? Constant exposure to loud noises isn't just annoying—it can contribute to stress-related illnesses over time. High noise levels are linked to issues like sleep disturbances and cardiovascular problems.

To combat this, find moments of quiet in your day. Creating a serene space in your home where you can retreat helps maintain peace of mind. Additionally, using soundproofing solutions like curtains or carpets reduces noise levels indoors.

Light Exposure

The type of light you're exposed to matters too! Natural sunlight is fantastic since it helps our bodies synthesize vitamin D but be careful with too much sun exposure—always wear sunscreen outdoors.

Conversely, blue light from screens before bed can interfere with sleep patterns by disrupting melatonin production in our brains. Experts recommend reducing screen use two hours before bedtime or using 'night mode' features on gadgets to limit exposure.

ENVIRONMENTAL FACTOR	TIPS FOR IMPROVEMENT
Air	Use indoor plants; track local air quality
Water	Filter tap water; check local quality reports
Food	Choose organic; read labels carefully
Noise	Designate a quiet home area; soundproof
Light	Limit screen time before bed; sunscreen outdoors

By understanding these basic environmental influences on health, you take essential steps toward preventing disease and supporting long-term wellness. Every small change brings us closer to living a healthier life amidst environmental challenges. With awareness and proactive measures, leveraging nature's offerings becomes second nature on this journey towards optimal health.

CHAPTER 10
LIFESTYLE FOR OPTIMAL MITOCHONDRIAL HEALTH

Exercise Routines

It's no secret that exercise is good for you. We've all heard it before: staying active keeps the heart healthy, the mind sharp, and the body fit. But when it comes to taking care of our mitochondria, our body's little powerhouses, exercise takes on a new level of importance.

Regular physical activity can boost the number and efficiency of mitochondria in your cells. Think of exercise as a tune-up for these tiny engines, improving their ability to generate energy effectively. But not all exercises are created equal when it comes to mitochondrial benefits.

There are primarily two types of exercises that play a crucial role in mitochondrial health: aerobic (or cardio) exercises and resistance training.

1. **Aerobic Exercises:** These include activities like running, cycling, swimming, and brisk walking. Aerobic exercise increases your heart rate and breathing rate significantly, which promotes better oxygen use by the cells. Over time, aerobic workouts can enhance the ability of mitochondria to produce energy. This type of exercise is particularly effective at increasing mitochondrial volume—meaning more energy producers in your muscle cells.

2. **Resistance Training:** Resistance exercises involve activities like weight lifting or using resistance bands. While it's commonly known for building muscle strength, it's also beneficial for maintaining mitochondrial function as we age. Studies have shown that resistance training can help stimulate muscle protein synthesis and improve the quality of existing mitochondria.

To reap maximum benefits for mitochondrial health, it's essential to incorporate both aerobic and resistance exercises into your routine.

WEEKLY EXERCISE BLUEPRINT:

Monday: 30 minutes of brisk walking + 20 minutes core strengthening exercises

Tuesday: Rest or gentle yoga

Wednesday: 45 minutes cycling or swimming + 15 minutes upper body strength training

Thursday: Rest or light stretching

Friday: 30 minutes jogging + 20 minutes lower body workout

Saturday: group fitness class or a recreational sport like tennis

Sunday: Complete rest or light nature walk

Remember, consistency is key—as little as 30 minutes per day can make a significant difference over time. Below is a simple chart illustrating how different exercises affect mitochondrial efficiency over time:

EXERCISE TYPE	SHORT TERM EFFECTS	LONG TERM EFFECTS
Aerobic	Improved oxygen consumption	Increased mitochondrial volume
Resistance	Polished protein synthesis	Enhanced mitochondrial function in aging muscles

While pushing yourself during workouts is beneficial, it's crucial to stay within healthy limits. Overtraining without adequate rest can stress your body and affect mitochondrial health adversely. Listening to your body when it requires some quiet time is crucial; adequate rest allows for recovery which is vital as well.

Exercise doesn't just fortify your physique; it's also essential nourishment for those microscopic engines powering every cellular function. An optimal blend of cardio and strength training stimulates growth and efficient working within your cells' mitochondria—leading you towards overall vitality!

Reducing Oxidative Stress

Our body's cells generate energy. During this process, they produce reactive molecules called free radicals. These are like the wild party crashers in your cells—they can cause damage if left unchecked. To keep them in line, our body uses antioxidants. It's a bit like having a good security team at that wild party, ensuring things don't get out of control.

The root of oxidative stress lies in balance—or imbalance—between these free radicals and antioxidants. When we have an overload of free radicals without enough antioxidants to neutralize them, that's when oxidative stress occurs. Over time, this can wear down our cells, including those powerhouse mitochondria we've been talking about.

So how do we reduce oxidative stress? Let's break it down into easy-to-grab tips:

1. **Hydrate Wisely:** Water isn't just a thirst-quencher; it's vital for detoxifying your body. Staying well-hydrated supports the body's natural ability to flush out toxins.
2. **Eat the Rainbow:** We've touched on nutrition before, but let's dive deeper into antioxidants like vitamin C (oranges), vitamin E (almonds), and beta-carotene (carrots). A colorful plate isn't just visually pleasing—it's packing a protective punch against oxidative stress.
3. **Green Tea Time:** Swap one of your usual drinks for green tea now and then. It's rich in catechins, powerful antioxidants that help fend off those unchecked party crashers—er, free radicals.
4. **Spice Things Up:** Incorporating spices like turmeric, which contains curcumin, provides anti-inflammatory and antioxidant effects. It's an easy add-on to soups or curries.
5. **Wine Wisely:** Moderate consumption of red wine brings resveratrol to the mix—a beneficial antioxidant known for its heart-healthy benefits. Remember, moderation is key!
6. **Mindful Breathing:** Sounds simple? It is! Deep breathing exercises reduce stress hormones that can otherwise accelerate oxidative damage in the body.
7. **Protective Environment:** Limit exposure to pollution by opting for indoor plants like spider plants or peace lilies; they're great at filtering indoor air pollutants.
8. **Adequate Sleep:** Sleep is when your body gets its repair work done, undoing much of the day's oxidative stress accumulation—another reason not to skimp on those ZZZs!

Implementing these tips may seem small individually but together have a profound cumulative effect on mitochondrial resilience against oxidative stress—not unlike how tiny sparks light up immense bonfires when combined!

Long-Term Care for Aging

As we gracefully move along the journey of life, taking care of our mitochondria becomes more important than ever. These tiny powerhouses are responsible for fueling every cell in our body, so understanding how to maintain their health is crucial for long-term vitality and aging gracefully. Fortunately, fostering optimal mitochondrial health doesn't have to be overwhelming. Let's explore some straightforward strategies that can enrich your life and keep you thriving well into your golden years.

Embracing a Balanced Sleep Routine

One of the cornerstones of maintaining healthy mitochondria as we age is getting adequate sleep. Our bodies repair themselves during sleep, and this includes mitochondrial rejuvenation. Aim for 7 to 9 hours of quality sleep per night. Setting a consistent sleep schedule by going to bed and waking up at the same time each day can work wonders in regulating your body's internal clock. Creating a relaxing bedtime routine, such as reading or taking a warm bath, can also improve sleep quality.

Managing Stress with Relaxation Techniques

Chronic stress can take a toll on mitochondrial health, leading to decreased function over time. Incorporating relaxation techniques into your daily routine can help mitigate stress and support mitochondrial longevity. Practices such as meditation, deep breathing exercises, or even listening to calming music can effectively reduce stress levels. Spending time outdoors and connecting with nature is another natural way to unwind and refresh your mind.

Hydration: A Key Component

Staying hydrated is crucial, especially as we grow older. Proper hydration supports cellular functions, including those carried out by mitochondria. It helps transport nutrients and remove waste products, which is essential for maintaining healthy cells. Make it a habit to drink water throughout the day—keeping a refillable bottle handy can serve as a helpful reminder.

Nurturing Social Connections

Engaging in social activities and nurturing relationships have been shown to have positive effects on overall health and well-being. Regular interaction with friends and family not only boosts your mood but also influences physical health positively, including mitochondrial efficiency. Whether it's joining clubs, attending social events, or simply having regular catch-ups with loved ones over coffee or tea—these interactions are beneficial for both mental and mitochondrial health.

Embracing New Hobbies

Learning new skills or engaging in hobbies is excellent for brain health and keeps your mind sharp as you age—a boon for mitochondrial activity too! Consider picking up a new hobby like painting, gardening, or learning an instrument; these encourage mental stimulation and satisfaction, contributing positively to cellular energy production.

Monitoring Your Mitochondrial Wellness

While we've touched on routine health screenings earlier in this book, it's worth emphasizing the importance of keeping tabs on your mitochondrial wellness specifically. This might involve discussions with healthcare professionals about blood tests that look at markers of oxidative stress or cellular energy production. Staying informed about your mitochondrial health will allow you to make necessary lifestyle adjustments promptly.

Regularly reassessing these habits ensures you're adapting optimally as life progresses. Embrace these practices not just as lifestyle adjustments but as enjoyable facets of nurturing lifelong vitality through mitochondrial care.

Avoiding Toxins and Harmful Habits

Living a lifestyle geared toward optimal mitochondrial health means considering what we allow into our bodies and environments. Our mitochondria, essential for powering our cells, are vulnerable to various environmental toxins and harmful habits that can impede their function.

We encounter potential toxins in our daily lives, from household cleaners to air pollution. Reducing exposure starts at home by choosing natural or non-toxic cleaning products. Many conventional cleaners contain volatile organic compounds (VOCs), which can hamper mitochondrial function when inhaled. Alternatively, simple solutions like vinegar and baking soda can effectively clean without toxic residues.

Another important consideration is what we put in and on our bodies. Pesticides present on non-organic produce are another common source of toxin exposure. Whenever possible, choose organic fruits and vegetables to lessen the pesticide load on your body. Similarly, opt for skincare products free of parabens, phthalates, and synthetic fragrances, as these ingredients sometimes include chemicals that your mitochondria dislike.

It's also essential to be mindful of heavy metals like lead and mercury. These elements can accumulate in the body over time from sources such as contaminated water or certain fish high in mercury. Consuming fish lower on the food chain such as sardines or herring can limit mercury intake while still providing beneficial omega-3 fats.

Additionally, it's crucial to consider the role of plastics in our everyday lives. Plastics can leach harmful chemicals like bisphenol A (BPA) into our food and water, potentially disrupting mitochondrial health. Use glass or stainless steel containers for food storage and choose BPA-free products when possible.

Smoking, excessive alcohol consumption, and drug use should also be avoided due to their well-documented detrimental effects on cellular health, including mitochondrial impairment. Quitting smoking drastically improves not just lung health but also boosts the efficiency of mitochondria throughout the body.

Consider your environment's impact on your well-being too. Indoor pollution sources such as poor ventilation or mold can be insidious threats to mitochondrial health. Investing in a quality HEPA air filter can ensure cleaner indoor air quality.

Even something as simple as limiting unnecessary medication use is beneficial for reducing toxin load on your mitochondria. While necessary medications should never be avoided without consulting a physician, being aware of potential overconsumption allows you to make informed decisions about what's truly necessary for your health journey.

CATEGORY	COMMON TOXIN/PRODUCT	SAFER ALTERNATIVE
Household Cleaners	VOCs-based sprays	Vinegar + Baking Soda
Produce	High-pesticide fruits	Organic options
Skincare	Parabens/Phthalates	Natural ingredient brands
Cookware/Food Storage	Plastic containers	Glass/Stainless Steel
Seafood	Shark/Tuna (high mercury)	Sardines/H meringue (low mercury)

In this way, by consciously choosing what we expose ourselves too - in both our diets and environments - we provide our mitochondria with a supportive environment where they could thrive amidst ever-present modern-day challenges!

Mental And Emotional Wellness

Our emotional state intricately influences our physical health, particularly the efficiency and vitality of our mitochondria. One key factor affecting both mental wellness and mitochondrial function is stress. When we experience stress, our body enters a "fight or flight" mode, releasing hormones like cortisol that prepare us to face immediate challenges. However, chronic stress means prolonged exposure to these hormones, which can overwhelm the body's natural systems, including mitochondria.

Moreover, high stress levels can lead to increased oxidative stress—a condition where harmful molecules damage cells, including their mitochondria. Therefore, managing stress is crucial for preserving mitochondrial health.

Mindfulness meditation is a highly effective technique for mitigating stress. By focusing on your breath or a specific mantra, you can calm your mind and reduce cortisol levels. This practice not only helps in lowering stress but also enhances emotional resilience, thereby benefiting both your mind and mitochondria. Additionally, consider incorporating yoga or tai chi into your routine. Both practices blend physical movement with mental focus and deep breathing, offering a holistic approach to reduce stress.

Emotional well-being thrives on meaningful connections with others. Positive relationships foster support and understanding, contributing immensely to one's mental health. An emotionally balanced life nurtures an environment where mitochondria can function optimally.

Make it a habit to spend time with loved ones, whether through shared meals or walks in nature. Engaging in fulfilling conversations not only enriches life but also alleviates feelings of isolation that can lead to emotional distress.

Adopting a positive outlook on life has tangible benefits for mitochondrial function. Studies have shown that optimism correlates with reduced inflammation—another culprit linked with mitochondrial dysfunction.

Start by practicing gratitude daily; reflect on things you are thankful for each evening. Not only will this shift your mindset towards positivity, but it will also create a healthier internal environment supportive of vibrant mitochondria.

Sleep quality significantly impacts mental wellness. During sleep, your brain processes emotions and repairs itself from daily wear—processes essential for maintaining cognitive function and mood stability. Aim for 7-9 hours of quality sleep per night to ensure optimal brain health and efficient mitochondrial function. Develop a calming pre-sleep routine; limit screen time an hour before bed as blue light disrupts the production of melatonin, a hormone crucial for sleep regulation.

Developing emotional resilience—the ability to bounce back from adversity—is key to protecting your mental health under strain. Techniques such as cognitive-behavioral strategies can help you reinterpret challenges positively rather than letting them drain your energy. By boosting resilience, we foster an adaptable spirit that upholds mental wellness and mitigates the impact of stress on mitochondria.

Don't underestimate the power of joy in supporting mitochondrial health! Engage in activities that bring happiness—be it painting, playing music, gardening, or watching comedies. Such endeavors stimulate dopamine production (the "feel-good" neurotransmitter), enhancing mood while encouraging efficient mitochondrial performance.

CONCLUSION

As we draw to the close of our exploration into the world of mitochondrial health and the remarkable benefits of methylene blue, it's essential to reflect on what we've uncovered and its impact on our lives. Mitochondrial health is fundamentally crucial because mitochondria are the powerhouses of our cells, responsible for producing the energy we need to function efficiently. When mitochondrial health is compromised, it can lead to a wide array of diseases and health conditions, affecting everything from your brain to your heart.

Mitochondrial dysfunction has been linked with neurodegenerative diseases like Alzheimer's and Parkinson's, metabolic disorders such as diabetes, and cardiovascular diseases. It's also been associated with immune system deficiencies and mental health issues. Therefore, maintaining optimal mitochondrial function isn't just about addressing existing health issues; it's about preventing a plethora of potential future problems.

Enter methylene blue—a compound with a rich history and promising potential in revolutionizing how we approach treatment for these dysfunctions. Its ability to improve mitochondrial efficiency means it can be a powerful ally in pursuing lifelong well-being. The research into methylene blue shows that it may enhance cellular respiration and offer neuroprotective effects, amongst other benefits. This makes it a compelling addition to your health regimen when used responsibly.

However, integrating methylene blue into daily life isn't about abandoning all other health protocols or viewing it as a cure-all. Instead, it's about understanding its role as part of a broader strategy for health maintenance and disease prevention. By incorporating methylene blue thoughtfully—perhaps under medical guidance—you give yourself an additional tool in the arsenal for maintaining robust mitochondrial function.

This knowledge brings us to one of the most empowering messages from this journey: you have significant control over your health. Making proactive choices in your daily routines—whether through diet, exercise, stress management, or supplementation with substances like methylene blue—can profoundly impact your overall well-being.

Remember that while science continues to unveil groundbreaking insights yearly; fundamental aspects like balanced nutrition, regular physical activity, adequate rest, and mindfulness remain just as vital. By harmonizing these traditional tenets of good health with new discoveries such as those related to methylene blue, you position yourself not only for longevity but for a quality life brimming with energy and vitality.

The challenge now lies in taking decisive steps towards nourishing your mitochondria and molding lifestyle choices that align with long-term wellness goals. You hold the power to shape your destiny concerning personal health outcomes by fostering an environment that supports cellular energy proliferation and diminishes unnecessary stressors or toxins.

So, embracing every opportunity for improvement—knowing that each decision steers you toward thriving at any age. Here's to unlocking not just longer life but better life through empowered action fueled by knowledge compiled within these pages!

Made in the USA
Las Vegas, NV
12 February 2025